Patient or Pawn?

Epic fails in health care, the approaching perfect storm and strategies for self-preservation

Jo Kline, J.D.

Patient or Pawn?

Epic fails in health care,
the approaching perfect storm
and strategies for self-preservation

Jo Kline, J.D.

Published in the United States of America by
Providentia Publishing
West Des Moines, Iowa

ISBN Print Edition: 978-0-578-94061-8
(available in e-book edition at Amazon.com)

www.JoKline.net

Book cover design by Jo Kline.

Just to be clear: This is *not* a book about COVID-19

I started writing *Patient or Pawn?* quite awhile before the term *COVID-19* had even been uttered. By the time I finished, the pool of knowledge about this coronavirus remained fairly shallow, but at least we had begun to know what we didn't know—and that's more important than you may now realize. Looking back at the early days of the pandemic, it's alarming to see how effortlessly this plague limited access to health care, stole rights to disclosure and consent and disregarded autonomy at life's end. Just like that.

We got a reality check on how little we know about being informed and safe health care consumers. *Which information sources are reliable? Is my risk for this disease greater than for other people? How can I preserve my rights as a patient in an emergency?* As COVID-19 took its greatest toll on the aging and those with chronic conditions, it underscored the critical issue of comorbidity in America and pulled back the curtain on health care inequities. Systemic weaknesses in research, logistics and technology became all too apparent, along with consumers' failure to be health literate. Soon enough, dysfunctional communication between policy makers and constituents was more than just an annoyance. For many it became *life-limiting,* an incurable condition that ultimately threatens one's survival. In this book, you will come to recognize well-established patterns in how health care is overseen in America, and you will better understand why the response to this pandemic was so chaotic. In many ways, how politicians, bureaucrats, stakeholders and clinicians managed the spread of COVID-19 was a dress rehearsal for the health care calamity that still lies ahead.

Of two things you can be certain: Whether facing a global pandemic, a perfect storm of health care access or a personal medical emergency, the challenges of decision making and care management remain the same. But unlike a pandemic, the arrival of the approaching perfect storm will be stealth and clandestine. You may not even notice we've reached critical mass until *you* are the one needing an appointment or an MRI or an ambulance. And the imminent perfect storm of health care promises to be of much greater intensity and duration than COVID-19, so fasten your seat belt.

Other books by Jo Kline, J.D.

THE 60-MINUTE GUIDE
TO HEALTH LITERACY
A common sense approach to
informed medical decision making

The practical guide to
Health Care Advance Directives
(2015)

EXIT – A novel about dying

SO GROWS THE TREE
Creating an Ethical Will
The legacy of your beliefs and values,
life lessons and hopes for the future

The Workshop Edition of
SO GROWS THE TREE

Whose big idea was that?
Lessons in giving from the
pioneers of value-inspired philanthropy

Last things first, just in case...
The practical guide to Living Wills
and Durable Powers of Attorney for Health Care
(2006)

Principles of Tax-deferred Exchanging
(1996 and 2001 editions)

ACRONYMS

ACA - Affordable Care Act of 2010
ACF - Administration for Children and Families
ACL - Administration for Community Living (fka Administration on Aging, the Office on Disability, and the Administration on Developmental Disabilities)
ADE - Adverse drug events
ADR - Adverse drug reactions
AHRQ - Agency for Healthcare Research and Quality
CDC - Centers for Disease Control and Prevention
CMS - Centers for Medicare & Medicaid Services
COGME - Council on Graduate Medical Education
DPC - Direct primary care
ED - Emergency Department
EHR - Electronic health record
FDA - U.S. Food and Drug Administration
GMENAC - Graduate Medical Education National Advisory Committee
HAC - Hospital-acquired condition
HAI - Healthcare-associated infection, aka Hospital-acquired infection
HHS - U.S. Department of Health and Human Services
HITECH - Health Information Technology for Economic and Clinical Health Act
HL7 - Health Level Seven International
HPSA - Health Professional Shortage Areas
HRSA - Health Resources and Services Administration
IOM - Institute of Medicine (nka National Academy of Medicine)
MACPAC - Medicaid and CHIP Payment and Access Commission
MedPAC - Medicare Payment Advisory Commission
NCHWA - National Center for Health Workforce Analysis
NHCWC - National Health Care Workforce Commission
NIH - National Institutes of Health
NP - Nurse practitioner
ODPHP - Office of Disease Prevention and Health Promotion
ONC - Office of the National Coordinator for Health Information Technology
PCMH - Patient-centered medical home
PA - Physician assistant
PCP - Primary care provider
PPRC - Physician Payment Review Commission
PSDA - Patient Self-Determination Act
VHA - Veterans Health Administration

TABLE OF CONTENTS

PART ONE 1
What in the world is going on?

CHAPTER ONE 3
We find ourselves on the horns of a dilemma

CHAPTER TWO 13
That was then and this is not then

CHAPTER THREE 23
The first element of the perfect storm

CHAPTER FOUR 31
The second element of the perfect storm

CHAPTER FIVE 47
The third element of the perfect storm

CHAPTER SIX 51
No worries. They've got this.

PART TWO 61
Where does this leave us?

CHAPTER SEVEN 63
What happens when you take it personally

CHAPTER EIGHT 69
How health care professionals are prepping

CHAPTER NINE 77
Lessons in how *not* to raise health literacy

PART THREE 87
Strategies for self-preservation

CHAPTER TEN 89
Aim to be at the table, not on the menu

CHAPTER ELEVEN **93**
Health Literacy: The secret ingredient
Strategies for self-preservation / Health literacy **94**

CHAPTER TWELVE **97**
Try really hard not to be invisible
Strategies for self-preservation / Being visible **101**

CHAPTER THIRTEEN **105**
Death: The ultimate adverse event
Strategies for self-preservation / Medical errors **113**

CHAPTER FOURTEEN **117**
Technology and the digital age
Strategies for self-preservation / Electronic health records **126**
Strategies for self-preservation / Telehealth **130**
Strategies for self-preservation / Telemedicine **134**
Strategies for self-preservation / Diagnostics & treatment **137**
Strategies for self-preservation / Technology & medical errors **139**

CHAPTER FIFTEEN **141**
Medication and polypharmacy
Strategies for self-preservation / Medication & polypharmacy **146**

CHAPTER SIXTEEN **149**
Care management and handoffs
Strategies for self-preservation / Care management & handoffs **153**

A FEW CLOSING REMARKS **157**

ENDNOTES **161**

ABOUT THE AUTHOR **204**

PART ONE

What in the world is going on?

CHAPTER ONE

We find ourselves on the horns of a dilemma

When a storm approaches, you have two alternatives: make a run for it or shelter in place. However, if that dark cloud on the horizon is destined to impact every facet of health care access and delivery, heading for the hills isn't a viable option. You must decide whether to remain a pawn amid a systemic meltdown or be an empowered patient armed with strategies for self-preservation. The time to choose is now.

No, it is not just you

Stop me if you've heard these. A 67-year-old man learns he has advanced prostate cancer. Once the urologist explains all the likely risks and benefits and makes his recommendation, the patient gives consent for a prostatectomy. He accepts the potential dangers and side effects in the belief he's making a fully informed and prudent decision, considering his diagnosis. There's just one hitch in that line of thinking: The diagnosis isn't his. As he discovers *after* the surgery, his original biopsy showed a normal and cancer-free prostate. The pathologist's bar code scanner detected the wrong form in a stack of papers, inadvertently switching the patient's records with those of another man who really does have cancer. A simple, life-altering digital technology snafu.

The second setting is a hospital emergency department (ED). A patient arrives by ambulance with signs of cardiac distress, and emergency personnel receive a copy of his health care advance directive, a Living Will. After considering his medical condition and wishes to forego life-prolonging measures, the vast majority of health care professionals in this situation skip lifesaving procedures and focus solely on keeping the patient comfortable. Why? Because they mistakenly think a Living Will is the same as a do-not-resuscitate order (DNR) that they believe—also mistakenly—directs them to simply provide comfort care. Luckily, this patient was a fictitious subject for research purposes only.

Disturbing, but both stories are true.[1] Perhaps you or someone close to you has had a similar experience. For me, it was a textbook case of patient-provider miscommunication in 2016 that brought me to this place. Even though I had written two books on Advance Care Planning, when confronted with a health care situation requiring shared decision making, it turns out I wasn't *health literate*. I quickly got motivated to fix that before the next medical crisis came along. Guess what I discovered—there were no available resources to guide me in becoming an informed decision maker. I dug in and learned all there is to know about health literacy, but it was just the start of uncovering what threatens our access to appropriate and safe health care.

First, whenever I spoke about my own experience, others told me how they had also felt confused and overwhelmed in health care situations. Some had even suffered unintended harm. Their stories were troubling and, eventually, all too common. Second, after hitting that speed bump in my journey, I did even more research on America's health care demographics and found startling evidence of what's already happening and about to get much worse. But you know, whenever I shared those revelations with a policy maker or health care stakeholder, their response was disbelief.

I bet you've noticed subtle changes. Senior housing alternatives are popping up everywhere. A board-certified specialist you or a friend relied upon is suddenly gone and you're nudged to see a nurse practitioner (NP) or physician assistant (PA) instead. At times you've felt ignored or at a loss in a health care crisis, and maybe you've even thought, *Is it just me?* I'm here to tell you, it is not just you. The stories at the beginning of this chapter illustrate two elements of modern health care, technology and information overload, that can so easily jeopardize patient safety. They're also symptomatic of the approaching perfect storm.

This is not your grandparents' or even your parents' health care environment. Medical conditions and treatment options have grown in variety and complexity; our beliefs and attitudes about health care have shifted; the patient-provider relationship is changing; and the nature of lifestyles and personal relationships is in flux. If you're thinking, *But it seems like there's something more going on*, you're absolutely right, grasshopper. And that *something* is why there's a sense of urgency in preparing for what's coming.

Auntie Em! Auntie Em!

There was no warning. In August of 2020, we had a cataclysmic weather event in Iowa that has never before happened and we hope like hell never does again. We experienced a *derecho*, the equivalent of a Category 4 inland hurricane and it was the most costly thunderstorm in modern U.S. history. With winds of 70 to 140 miles per hour sustained for 30 to 45 minutes, it completely freaked me out—and I've been through a lot of tornado near-misses. We had no concept of its power until it was over: the death of three Iowans, a statewide decimation of our tree canopy, $8 billion in property losses and the damage or destruction of over six million acres of corn and soybeans—nearly one third of Iowa's crops. No derecho alarm had sounded, no hint of what was about to happen.

Thankfully, the perfect storm of health care brewing just over America's horizon isn't like that. You will learn there are all kinds of warning signs. In *Patient or Pawn?*, we'll start with demographics, where it is obvious that 70 years after a baby boom, there's going to be an elder boom. Duh. Furthermore, the patients now sidling their way into the system in high numbers are not your average health care consumers. Oh no. They're the frequent fliers of medicine. Some are older, but most are people of all ages with chronic or complex diseases. Chapter Three has astonishing figures that shed light on the systemic pressures you're already sensing.

Then consider this: Baby Boomers are not just aging into the system as patients, they're also aging out as health care professionals. We know quite a lot about what health care demands and supplies will look like in the coming decades, both in the labor force and in hard dollar costs. In Chapter Four you'll see that America's aging trajectory doesn't level off until 2060—it's like a derecho that hangs around for days instead of minutes. With all its fury, there is no question the perfect storm of health care will mean delays for *everyone* in accessing medical diagnostics and treatments.

As we follow the history of what Baby Boomers have met at each stage of life, you'll realize the current denial and lack of preparedness are nothing new. What makes this phase so different? Postponing health care has potentially tragic implications, certainly when compared to the disappointment of being on a waiting list for a VW Beetle. This new chapter in the Boomers' lives is a potential disaster for *every* American trying to access timely and competent health care. For Boomers, it's déjà vu all over again. Here we are, once more knocking at the door—as we have so many times throughout our lives—and hearing *Where did you all come from?* It's simple, really: *Demography is destiny.*[2] You can use the most sophisticated forecasting simulation models known to man and you will not be as confident as I am of this: *Ten years from now, every one of today's 55-year-olds will either be 65 or dead.*

I'll use health care's complex statistics to show how macro demographics and economics impact us as individuals, and then I'll share how to use that knowledge to preserve your rights and to protect those you care about. Throughout the pages of *Patient or Pawn?* you'll witness the unavoidable collision of 1) demographics, 2) dwindling resources and 3) consumers' lack of health literacy, and you'll see how this perfect storm is turning traditional health care delivery on its ear. Why should you care about the scheduling and staffing challenges already plaguing clinics, laboratories and hospitals if you're not at least age 57 or have a chronic condition? Because at some point you will face these issues yourself or as a loved one's advocate. Preserving a patient's rights in medical decision making is already a formidable responsibility, even without 330 million others vying for access to the same health care resources.

Hey, who made this mess?

As you begin to appreciate the impending threats to health care access, you might be asking yourself, *Who let this happen?* Let's start with everyone who has demanded and benefited from medical advances in diagnostics, treatments and cures; those who have largely ignored demographic realities; and anyone whose only goal was to achieve the highest revenue at the lowest cost. The simple answer to the question *Who let this happen?* is *Practically everyone.* Patients, providers, policy makers, bureaucrats and stakeholders have all worked in unison to create a Frankenstein-ish health care system now turning on its master. And how well America anticipates and ultimately prepares for what's coming is as significant as any medical condition you'll ever experience.

Right about now, you may also be wondering if you're the last person to learn what's in store for health care in America. I doubt very much you are, but if you haven't heard much about it before, maybe that's because nearly all stakeholders and policy makers (and candidates to become policy makers) are of two schools: 1) those who don't know it or 2) those who don't want *you* to know it. It begs the question: *What have the real change agents of health care been doing to gather valuable intel and make preparations for this perfect storm? Patient or Pawn?* answers that, and you'll also get a glimpse at how some providers are reinventing health care delivery. You may or may not be crazy about what they're up to.

By the time you've finished Parts One and Two, the severity and certainty of the arising crisis will be clear. When we get to Part Three, you will be more than ready to learn strategies to become an informed decision maker and care manager. I hope you will come to believe—as I already do—that each and every one of us has the innate power to master the skills and tools of self-preservation, despite imminent challenges. Powers just waiting to be tapped.

My mission is most assuredly not to rescue the flailing health care system as it now exists, and I don't have a miraculous reform package up my sleeve. *Patient or Pawn?* exposes the circumstances threatening your timely access to health care and the attitudes and practices now steering American health care away from its true mission. Most importantly, here you will find strategies to preserve personal rights to informed consent, autonomy and safety. But *Patient or Pawn?* does not advance any one systemic solution. I am concerned only with giving you practical action steps and reason to hope that with the right preparation, you and those you advocate for will have the best health outcomes until natural death occurs. And sooner or later it will.

This is what a winner looks like

You will see that although *self-preservation* doesn't always result in *survival*, it can be equally significant. Self-preservation is remaining an autonomous and safe patient to the very end of your journey. What does it take to achieve it? While we cannot alter inescapable demographics and a dwindling supply of health care resources, left standing is the third element of this perfect storm, Americans' pervasive lack of health literacy.

Being health literate is recognizing when, how and where to access, process and understand basic health information and services needed to make informed decisions. It is the one component in our exclusive control as individuals, and its information-gathering and decision-making skills will make the most efficient use of whatever health care resources are available. In this game, being health literate is what it takes to achieve self-preservation, what it takes to be a winner.

Let's face it, humans are not born judicious decision makers. It hasn't helped that throughout health care's evolution, it's never been the priority of policy makers or stakeholders or even practitioners to guide patients in health literate decision making, though we've known how to do that for some time now. As a result—and this is where most people find themselves—we're lousy at making informed choices. I truly believe that's only because we haven't been offered the skills and tools to be engaged health care consumers. Whatever the reason behind our blissful ignorance until now, we can no longer afford to remain that way.

Anytime a critical demand confronts a limited supply of resources, there are going to be winners and losers. *Patient or Pawn?* is about the system's questionable capacity to meet your predictable health care needs. This is a game with very high stakes—life itself. As you heed each caution and master each strategy contained here, you are one step closer to being the empowered patient and advocate you deserve to be, and *must* be for self-preservation. One step closer to being a winner.

Okay, here's the plan

Effective decision making is key to achieving the best health outcomes possible, no matter how short or long one's life may be. As you will learn in Chapter Five, we have oodles of studies on Americans' big fail at being informed decision makers. For the most part, researchers conclude we are not capable of being fully engaged and participating partners in our health care. Yes, they actually say that. As a result, their recommendations focus on dumbing down patient-provider communication. Practically speaking, that has meant encouraging doctors to use smaller words (and bigger print), avoid medical terms and limit the information they share in communicating with us. That doesn't really work for me and I wouldn't recommend it for you, either. Rather than lowering expectations for patients' level of engagement in care management, the best way to overcome low health literacy is to elevate decision-making skills—on both sides of the provider-patient relationship. I say we try using all that health literacy research to improve access, foster patient safety and achieve better health outcomes.

What if you could approach health care management and decision making with confidence, sensing potential hazards lying ahead and having the skills and processes for an optimal experience, no matter what leaps into your path? You can. Grasping the strategies to win at this health care game determines whether you make informed decisions as an engaged patient or have the health care journey of someone else's choosing. Part Three includes straightforward action steps enabling you to:

- Understand the advantages of being health literate.
- Effectively access available health care resources.
- Act as an engaged advocate for yourself or someone else.
- Refuse to be an invisible health care consumer.
- Recognize, anticipate and avoid harmful medical errors.
- Be aware of the benefits and hazards of health care technology.
- Achieve the best health outcomes by being medication-savvy.
- Preserve patient safety with prudent care management and handoffs.

In an overcrowded health care system that fails to acknowledge and address known risks for end users, whether you recognize your rights and preserve them may well be a matter of life or death. Self-preservation requires patient empowerment, and every empowered patient must first be a health literate patient. Your choice.

Here's what I know about you

I do not believe there is a typical reader of this book. The personal and health care experiences motivating you are distinct from everyone else's. Still, I know quite a lot about you. I know:

- Odds are one in three you're a caregiver and/or substitute decision maker for someone else.
- There's a one in five chance you or a person close to you has already experienced a harmful medical error.
- You're inquisitive and resourceful when it comes to your health care.
- It's a flip of the coin whether you have two or more chronic medical conditions.
- You want to find and access appropriate and comprehensive health care for yourself and your loved ones.

As for that last item, whether you label it being *activated* or *health literate* or *engaged* or *empowered*, it means being a person with the information-gathering and decision-making skills and confidence to make fully informed health care choices.

By acknowledging and preparing for the approaching perfect storm of health care:

- You will be empowered and respected in health care situations.
- Your input and consent will be sought before any medical procedure.
- You will be a fully-participating partner in shared decision making.
- Your autonomy as an individual will be honored.

- You will have the best possible health outcomes.
- And this is a biggie—you are much more likely to remain safe on your health care journey, unharmed by a medical error.

Raise your hand if you've ever skipped to the last page of a book to see how the story ends. If you're tempted to do so after reading some of the unsettling statistics following here, let me assure you this story ends with *reason to hope*. There is *reason to hope* that by practicing simple strategies, you can preserve your rights to informed consent, autonomy and safety at any point along your health care journey. There is *reason to hope* that by taking health literacy action steps as an advocate, you can protect another person's rights as well. And there is *reason to hope* we can access available health care resources despite the challenges we face.

Here's what you should know about me

I have two confessions to make. First, I am not a health care professional. In fact, like you, I'm a health care consumer who frets over getting unexpected news I'm not ready to handle, such as learning of a life-limiting disease or—heaven forbid—that my doctor has stopped accepting Medicare reimbursement. I worry I won't have the presence of mind to fully absorb what I'm told and ask enough questions or any of the right ones. I don't dare to assume I'll always make prudent decisions. And even though I've got great Health Care Advance Directives (I drafted them), I fret about whether I'll have the end of life I want. As if that were something a human being could even plan in advance. Oh, I'm not done. I worry about not knowing what I'm fairly certain any ninth grader knows about the workings of the human body. Then, when I get a headache, a little part of me thinks it might be the first sign of a tumor. If I walk into a room and don't have a clue why, I wonder if it's the moment I will look back on as *when it all began*. A lot of you know what I'm talking about.

There is, however, something that sets me apart from most health care consumers and makes me uniquely qualified to write this book. It's not just that I'm a Baby Boomer and can attest firsthand to the demand/supply thing we've faced our entire lives. It's not just being an attorney, which anyone knows has little correlation with sound decision-making skills. And it's certainly not that I've figured it all out, although, not to brag, but I now know what I don't know. It's something even more personal.

Nearly 20 years ago when I began to learn, write and speak about medical decision making and what it means to have and be an effective health care advocate, I dealt exclusively with demographics and health care law surrounding incapacity and the end of life. Once my focus turned to health literacy, the stories I heard were of decision making crises all along the health care journey, and they stopped being second-hand tales. Instead, they began to feature my circle of friends and family—and me—as they encompassed the spectrum from infancy to end of life, from preventive care to hospice. Every day I am reminded of challenges inherent in the modern health care journey. So what makes me uncommonly prepared to tell this story is that I am *not* a health care professional. Like you, I came to this place through the patient portal. I just happen to be a health care consumer with a penchant for research and a passion to share with others what I discover.

That leads me to the second confession, which is that I am a recovering *pawn*. I first became interested in the law of medical decision making after observing the passing of two family members. One received palliative hospice care, one did not. It made me realize how little I knew about our rights to comfort, dignity and support at the end of life, as patients and as witnesses. From learning some important lessons more than once since then I know if I don't practice constant vigilance, I may slip up and unwittingly relinquish my rights as a patient and my safety along with them. In a flash. That thought can be very grounding.

Some housekeeping matters

I've tried to strike a balance between providing enough research detail to validate my assertions but not so much that it melts your mind. There are extensive citations in the Endnotes. You can confirm what I'm saying and dig even deeper if you choose. Throughout *Patient or Pawn?*, when I say "we" I mean health care consumers, whether that's direct end users, caregivers or substitute decision makers accessing information on behalf of others. And, I'll be honest, I'm hoping this book makes its way into the hands of some of the 15 million health care consumers who are also health care professionals. They fulfil their duties in an industry and culture that seldom acknowledge their daily commitment. Perhaps the information and perspectives provided here will make the journey a little smoother for them as healers, as well as patients. If only.

By the way, I've checked the readability score of this book. It's at an 11th grade level—five grades above the American Medical Association's recommendation for communicating with you. Personally, I think you can handle it.

What have you got to lose?

There has been an unwritten contract between patients and health care providers for a very long time. As free-thinking humans, we get to live as we choose, oblivious to the need for preventive care and potential health hazards and bothersome symptoms—unless, of course, they 1) refuse to be ignored or 2) the Internet can't provide an acceptable explanation and DIY treatment. From our perspective, implicit in this agreement is the health care provider's responsibility to successfully address our ailments and discover ways to handle little issues before they become big problems. Now, I'm sorry to be the one to carry this message, but it's time to put on our big people pants and become engaged participants in our health care. At this place and time in history, it's prudent to acknowledge that personal accountability is no longer optional if we want the best possible health outcomes to the end of life.

In any crisis, it's important to recognize what elements are in our control. If you look up and spot a tsunami on the horizon, it would be a profoundly poor use of your time to try to stop it. That can also be said of the approaching perfect storm of health care. These realities are not in question:

Truth #1. In the coming years and decades, more Americans will age and die than ever before in our history. A lot more.

Truth #2. It is magical thinking to believe the ordinary rules of supply and demand don't apply to health care resources. They really do.

Truth #3. Leaving your health care access and safety to chance—or in the hands of others—is folly. And dangerous.

Until now, every public conversation or debate about health care reform has involved all those claiming to act for the consumers of health care, folks such as major stakeholders, special interest groups, policy makers and bureaucrats. Hmm. Look who's not at the table: end users and their hands-on providers. The self-preservation strategies of *Patient or Pawn?* suggest some distinct advantages in having these two outlier groups join forces, hunker down and make health care truly work for those most directly impacted: patients and their clinicians. Would you like to get in on that? Good, because the alternative is not pretty. Over the next 24 hours:

- 10,000 more Americans will qualify to join Medicare.[3]
- 1,300 will be diagnosed with Alzheimer's disease.[4]
- 200 nurses will celebrate retirement.[5]

The forces coming together to create this perfect storm of health care in America are inevitable and easily recognized. But never confuse what's happening around us with how we choose to prepare for and react to it as individuals. The former is not in our control, the latter is. You and I and those we care about will face health care circumstances that hold no second chance to get it right, and the *need* to master strategies for self-preservation is clear. It is my fervent hope this book instills in you the *desire* to seek that path as well. I found my voice as a patient and so will you, if that's what you choose. What have you got to lose?

CHAPTER TWO

That was then and this is not then

For more than four decades, meager efforts to enhance the process of medical decision making have focused on Advance Care Planning with one goal in mind: Stop medicine from using life-prolonging measures to keep us alive against our wishes. Forty years of medical evolution have shown this 1976 model of decision making and care management to be dangerously narrow. And of little value on the health care journey of today.

The health care axis was shifted by three young women

I'm an attorney, so I'm not going to *not* talk about the role of law in health care access and delivery. There's no expectation for you to be familiar with the legal precedents of medical decision making and care management and no need. In the coming chapters, you will soon see the practical effects of not exercising one's rights as a patient and you will learn the simple action steps to preserve them. Still, please resist the temptation to skim over this part because you don't think you need to know legal stuff and/or because you have a preconceived notion the law is boring. You could not be more mistaken. First, understanding rights inherent in being an informed health care consumer is fundamental to having the best possible health outcomes. Second, at the heart of every legal dispute is a story of real people.

It was 1976 when the national media gave us our first up-close-and-personal glimpse at the medical profession's power to indefinitely prolong life with artificial means. We intruded unabashedly on a New Jersey family's struggle to make life-or-death decisions on behalf of their twenty-one-year-old daughter, Karen Ann Quinlan. She was in a persistent vegetative state, kept alive with a ventilator and feeding tube. After suing to be named her guardian, Karen Ann's father was given legal authority to choose whether to continue those life-prolonging measures. Once all the theological and ethical debates had been dealt with, the court's legal rationale left no doubt that, indeed, each of us has the right to first consent to any medical procedure, be it as ordinary as having one's blood pressure taken or as life-altering as the removal of a ventilator.[6]

Nature abhors a vacuum, and so does the law. The legislative knee-jerk reaction to *Quinlan* was to feverishly fill that bothersome void with a body of laws known as Advance Care Planning. This assortment of state and federal statutes is intended to guide the use of life-prolonging medical procedures for someone lacking decision making capacity if—and only if—triggered by the person's terminal illness or irreversible unconsciousness. Within a decade of *Quinlan,* the wildfire legislative movement resulted in a variety of Living Will and/or Durable Power of Attorney for Health Care statutes in three quarters of the states. The 1990 U.S. Supreme Court *Cruzan* case refined the legal issue of *what* we can decide on behalf of an incapacitated person in Missouri,[7] and by 1997, all 51 jurisdictions had weighed in with new laws. While it's true the 2005 *Schiavo* litigation in the Florida courts brought these questions once again front and center by focusing on *who* gets to decide,[8] lawmakers generally considered the issue of medical decision making to have already been well settled. Not so fast.

In their haste to jettison the threat of being kept alive against one's wishes, few had noticed Karen Ann Quinlan wasn't the fitting prototype for that ideology. As Karen Ann's mother said 20 years after her daughter's case had been decided, "*We never asked to have her die. We just asked to have her put back in a natural state so she could die in God's time.*"[9] Under the tenets of the Quinlans' Roman Catholic faith, a ventilator is an extraordinary means of treatment that may be removed under certain circumstances. Artificial nutrition is *not.* Which is why Karen Ann's father made the decision to keep the feeding tube in place once Karen Ann was weaned off the ventilator. She lived for another nine years in a vegetative state, the polar opposite of what those lawmakers presumably meant to happen in a similar situation.

Enter *patient autonomy,* a key element of medical decision making that got right past the lawmakers. Whether you would make the same decision as Mr. Quinlan is not relevant. Autonomy is exactly what sets us apart from each other and its role in medical decision making is absolute, even though noticeably absent from the Advance Care Planning laws sprouting up between 1976 and 1997. Every one of those statutes assumed, as many still do, that a person would *not* choose life-prolonging measures for himself or a loved one under triggering circumstances. Furthermore, health care and legal professionals (including me) were misguided in thinking there is no real need for health care decision-making skills until someone is nearly dead, or at least permanently asleep. We were wrong.

One of the principal purposes of statutes is to protect rights and liberties, and I'll leave to others the question of whether Advance Care Planning laws *ever* acted as autonomous and effective decision-making tools. They certainly don't provide the guidance needed in today's complex health care environment. Medical decision making is neither limited to the end of life nor exclusively age-centric, which makes this as good a time as any to identify America's *cohorts*, the groups of individuals having one or more demographic characteristics in common:

- Greatest Generation (born 1901 to 1927)
- Silent Generation (born 1928 to 1945)

- Baby Boom (born 1946 to 1964)
- Generation X (born 1965 to 1976, sometimes referred to as the Echo Boom)
- Millennial (born 1977 to 2000, sometimes referred to as Generation Y)
- Generation Z (born 2001 and after)
- Generation Alpha?

Over the past 40 years, we've traveled absurdly fast and come incredibly far in every facet of modern medicine. Somehow we've managed to do so without health care's end users ever learning how to be engaged and informed decision makers. That has to stop. First, when we try to manage health care with a narrow and outdated medical decision-making model, we find . . .

Medical conditions and treatment options have changed

To get a real sense of why navigating health care and medical decision making has become so complex and challenging, let's start with what kills us. In 1976, the top seven causes of death for Americans of all ages were:

1. Heart disease
2. Cancer
3. Stroke
4. Accidents
5. Influenza and pneumonia
6. Diabetes
7. Cirrhosis of the liver[10]

Compare that list to today's causes of death:

1. Heart disease
2. Cancer
3. Accidents
4. Respiratory diseases
5. Stroke
6. Alzheimer's disease
7. Diabetes[11]

We've knocked influenza and pneumonia down a few notches thanks to modern antibiotics, while the Hepatitis B vaccine and improved transfusion practices have dramatically reduced liver diseases, such as cirrhosis.[12] *Why haven't we made more advances in eradicating the biggest killers?* We have, and that's where part of the trouble begins. The two frontrunners for a very long time, heart disease (since 1910) and cancer (since 1933), now account for 44 percent of all deaths in America,[13] down 14 percent since 1976.[14] We've doubled the rate of survival from heart attacks, thanks to better diagnostics and emergency care, pharmacotherapy, a plethora of cardiac surgical procedures and reduced smoking (I still miss it).[15] That helped move heart disease from 38 percent to 23 percent of all deaths. Cancer's 5-year overall survival rate has risen 27 percent over the past three decades, and mortality from strokes has been reduced by one third during the same period.[16] So, while four of the seven deadliest diseases are hanging in there, they've certainly lost some of their steam.

Modern health care is keeping alive many who previously would not have survived an emergency or life-limiting medical condition. That has, in turn, caused extraordinary growth in one particular area of health care: *chronic illness*. We'll just ignore the intra-agency squabble at the Centers for Disease Control and Prevention (CDC) over the definition of a "chronic disease" (*three months or more* versus *one year or more*). A chronic disease requires ongoing medical attention or limits activities of daily living, or both, for an extended period of time.[17] However narrowly defined, the prevalence of chronic illness in America constitutes an epidemic.

Now, back to how a person's cause of death impacts their health care journey and rate of utilization. It depends on the *illness trajectory*, the pattern of declining health that ultimately ends in death. Chronic conditions, such as dementia and diabetes, have extended illness trajectories that can result in a protracted treatment path spanning years, maybe even decades. A sudden and unexpected passing, as caused by a massive stroke or heart attack, has a short vertical trajectory. Prolonged illness trajectories entail more intense and complex care management, increased use of providers, medications, procedures and caregiving services and the relentless decision making that comes with all of that.

In addition to six of the top seven causes of death (not accidents), the most common chronic illnesses are:

- Hypertension (high blood pressure)
- Hyperlipidemia (high cholesterol)
- Mood disorders (e.g., depression, anxiety, bipolar disorder)
- Upper respiratory disorders (e.g., sinus infections)
- Arthritis
- Asthma
- Sleep apnea
- Chronic kidney disease

Forty years ago, the chronic conditions of greatest frequency and most concern were hardening of the arteries, senility, stroke, mental disorders, arthritis, heart conditions and hypertension—the government's terms of art at the time. They affected fewer than 20 percent of all adults, and chronic illness for those under age 65 was a nonissue. Today, not so much. Most recent available statistics show 60 percent of *all* American adults, about 148 million of us, now have at least one chronic condition (*morbidity*).

Forty-two percent have two or more (*comorbidity*); and 12 percent have five or more chronic illnesses. (That last group has quadrupled in its share of adults since 2001.[18]) Unfortunately, 25 percent of children now also have at least one chronic condition.[19]

When someone requires health care management long before the end of life and that need continues for years, even decades, the decision-making model of Advance Care Planning. Doesn't. Work. The 1970s simplistic approach of *Triggering Event A, then Choice B* is no match for decisions surrounding the symptoms, diagnoses, side effects, lifestyle adaptations and caregiving needs of having one or more chronic conditions.

Besides being challenged by the changes in what ails and then kills us, health care management is also being tested by the complexity of prevention and care options now available. Our expectations are for treatments and cures to address all manner of medical issues, from little inconveniences to life-threatening emergencies. That adds up to information and decision-making overload, whether dealing with preventive care, an acute medical crisis or the long-term treatment of a chronic condition.

If overwhelmed by decision making, it might even be tempting to wish for fewer choices. Were we to travel not very far back in time, we would definitely have less to agonize over because now commonplace diagnostic and treatment options such as these did not yet exist: kidney dialysis, PET scans, CT scans, MRIs, joint replacements, ICDs and statins for high cholesterol. We've come to take these and similar therapies for granted and no one would wish it otherwise. But medical care should not be confused with health care management, and regrettably, what hasn't accompanied these medical advancements are the decision-making skills and tools they demand.

Chronic kidney disease (CKD) demonstrates how medical advances have complicated care management. We now have the diagnostics to detect CKD among the 37 million Americans estimated to have it, which means every year another 125,000 people face the option of whether to start dialysis and/or await a transplant. The 726,000 individuals currently on dialysis cope with daily care management choices regarding therapies, lifestyle changes, disease symptoms, treatment side effects and the additional chronic conditions that may accompany CKD, such as diabetes, heart disease and hypertension.[20] Kidney disease patients are among millions of Americans receiving unexpected diagnoses annually, news that prompts the need for critical decision making in both treating and managing an acute or chronic medical condition:

Diagnoses or events each year / The impact on patients' lives

- 805,000 heart attacks / 126.9 million living with heart disease[21]
- 900,000 new cases of congestive heart failure / 11 million cardiology visits[22]
- 795,000 strokes / 6 million living with potentially debilitating aftereffects[23]
- 1.3 million diabetes diagnoses / 34.2 million coping with diabetes[24]

- 1.8 million new cancer diagnoses / 16.9 million survivors on the watch[25]
- 93 million adults with high cholesterol / Increased risks for heart disease[26]

The traditional Advance Care Planning model is pathetically inadequate to address the challenges of managing treatment options; inherent risks and benefits; possible side effects; the advisability of a second opinion; the choice between curative measures, life-extending treatment or watchful waiting; and—always—the impact on the patient's overall well-being. Your ability to access needed information and services and achieve the best possible health outcomes is shaped largely by whether you have adequate decision-making skills. Because besides coping with the evolution in medical conditions and treatment options, when we try to manage health care with a narrow and outdated medical decision-making model, we also find that . . .

Our beliefs and attitudes have changed

As the 1976 *Quinlan* drama unfolded, the rallying cry "*It's wrong to keep the patient alive!*" led to two decades of remedial lawmaking, presumably reflective of prevailing public opinion. Fast forward 30 years and you could hear the crowds outside Theresa Schiavo's hospice chanting, "*It's wrong to let the patient die!*" Same situation with vastly different public sentiment being expressed. In their stark contrast, these divergent views illustrate *patient autonomy*—there it is again—which is decision making that incorporates personal beliefs, values and moral independence. Those qualities, as personified in each of us, are as unique as our fingerprints. Over the past four decades, we've changed as individuals and as a society. It happens. There's been a long, steep learning curve since 1976, but what has become all too obvious is that Advance Care Planning is not one size fits all.

Some evidence suggests we're moving further away from thinking a patient should sometimes be allowed to die and closer to believing we should always do everything possible to keep a patient alive.[27] At the same time, ten states have legalized physician-assisted suicide since 1997.[28] That's autonomy for you. These disparate positions prove the point: Lobbyists or special interest groups advocating for one policy or another to address theoretical medical dilemmas are irrelevant to those actually faced with a life-altering or life-limiting decision. That's when the pivot point of medical decision making should be the person vested with authority to grant autonomous consent. And that's when we find our time-worn decision-making model is ineffective for most of today's complex end-of-life choices, let alone acute medical crises or long-term chronic disease management.

Paternalism is the practice of proceeding without the patient's fully informed consent or acting contrary to the patient's wishes. It was the watchword of health care until not all that long ago. The patient might ultimately agree with the treatment plan, but under the paternalistic model of decision making, he has no role in granting consent. I will leave nameless the legal scholars and physician-journalists who assert a patient's right to informed consent has somehow been newly-fashioned in the past few decades, as they lament the demise of paternalistic medicine. They also seem to believe consent is a privilege being conferred by physicians, like passing an Olympic torch. Some even suggest "*unfettered patient autonomy is not necessarily a good thing*." Really? I'm no constitutional scholar, but I'm positive the 14th Amendment (the Touch-me-not Clause) granted due process and the implied right to privacy back in 1868.[29] Courts first affirmed the right to informed consent in medical care springing from the Constitution around the turn of the century—the one that began in 1900.[30] A patient's right to be fully informed about medical treatment and then to consent or refuse to consent or request withdrawal of treatment already begun has been around a very long time. Notwithstanding whether it is, on occasion, relinquished by patients and/or disregarded by providers.

The serious flaw lies in these experts' belief that respecting autonomous rights is a zero sum game: If the patient or proxy chooses and then advocates for a treatment plan, the provider no longer has a role in shaping the course of action. That's just wrongheaded and silly. It also presents an insurmountable hurdle for the health care consumer seeking to be part of a *shared* decision making health care team. Admittedly, having informed, empowered and free-thinking constituents was not among the goals of post-*Quinlan* lawmakers. Indeed, when access to information and options were both limited, it may have seemed more expedient for doctors or ethics committees to make the decisions, but today's patient knows stuff—lots of stuff.

- Health care consumers can now retrieve medical information even doctors couldn't easily access not long ago.
- There are more treatment alternatives to choose from and occasions requiring decision making than were ever imagined in the past.
- Possessing information does not equate to expertise and the health care provider is still the skilled professional in the room, even though teamed with a patient who has more data and choices than ever before.

It is both common sense and critical to integrate the provider's expertise and the patient's autonomy into shared decision making. The right to informed consent doesn't mean we're entitled to always have favorable choices—if only—but we do have a right to *autonomous* options that reflect our individual stories and treatment goals. Shared decision making demands an evolving patient-doctor relationship, and few among us are fully comfortable with our respective roles in this new mode of care management. That, my friend, is the problem. Health care choices have layers of complexity never contemplated in 1976, and maintaining autonomy while processing all that information is exhausting. All the same, the 1970s called and they want their medical decision-making model back.

Care management and decision making processes that don't embrace each patient's unique treatment and personal goals have no place in contemporary health care, but ever true is the maxim that if you want ten opinions on what constitutes "quality of life," just ask ten people. Besides coping with changes in medical conditions, treatment options and beliefs and attitudes, when we try to manage health care with a narrow and outdated medical decision-making model, we also find that . . .

Our lifestyles and personal relationships have changed

I loved growing up in the 1950s. Our post-war neighborhood was bursting with new homes and kids—lots of them. Every family had a garden, dads could fix most anything and the closest we came to *Stranger danger!* was to head for home when the streetlights came on. I once conducted a house-by-house census from memory and realized there were 33 children in 13 homes. I mean, I knew at the time there were a lot of us, but no way did I realize over half the people living in my 1965 neighborhood were under age 18. That soundly beat the national statistic of 37 percent.[31] There was not one single family in our hood that wasn't a mom, a dad and at least one child, the classic American *nuclear family* of the time.

How, where and with whom we live impacts health care management. What's the opposite of the archetypal nuclear family? The family of today. In 1950, 79 percent of households were headed by married couples; today it's less than half. The *number* of homes has more than doubled since the end of the Baby Boom, but the *size* of each household has shrunk by nearly an entire person.[32] Concerning access to care, it's significant that single-person households have grown from 9.3 percent in 1950 to 29 percent in 2019. Because we're able to keep folks alive and independent longer than ever before and because the divorce rate among seniors has tripled since 1990, more than four of every ten seniors now live alone.[33] Remember when it was major to turn 100? Not saying it still isn't, but you'd be joining 90,000 centenarians already living in the United States. By 2030, there will be 140,000. Nearly 600,000 by 2060.[34] You read that right.

What's the correlation between one's lifestyle and health care decision making? Crucial, if you're ever unable to think or speak for yourself. Unless you've experienced first-hand what happens when an incapacitated person doesn't have an appointed proxy and/or written care instructions, you may not realize each state specifies who can step in to make medical decisions. Decision making authority is granted to *surrogate decision makers.* Most states name the potential proxies and assign seniority as you would expect: spouse, adult child, parents, adult siblings. Those limited choices made perfect sense when these laws were fashioned. Now we're in a culture where Boomers had a birth rate 54 percent smaller than their Greatest Generation and Silent Generation parents, while the prevalence of unmarried adults has grown by 45 percent.[35] In fact, we already have labels for the one fifth of seniors with *no one* willing or able to advocate for them in a medical crisis: *elder orphans* and the *unbefriended.*[36] While several states have made laws more reflective of the modern "family," many still exclude a close friend, adult grandchild or domestic partner unless appointed as a health care proxy in writing prior to the patient's incapacity. Only one in four adults bothers to do that ahead of time.[37]

Yes, in theory, laws exist primarily to protect rights and liberties, but it is a goal not always met. Understandably, lawmakers of 40 years ago could not possibly foresee how soon and how thoroughly the changes in medical conditions, treatment options, beliefs, attitudes, lifestyles and relationships would render their statutory guidance irrelevant. The existing decision-making model offered up by health care's stakeholders and policy makers first assumes it won't even be needed until the last chapter of life, and second, that all health care consumers are of one mind. Wrong and wrong again. It is four decades behind the times. Other than that, it works just fine.

And if all that weren't enough . . .

Even though the United States and England profess to speak the same language, the Brits lay claim to many brilliant words we don't use nearly enough in the States. *Brilliant* is one. Another is *gobsmacked.* You can certainly say *utterly astonished* or *astounded*, but *gobsmacked* does a better job of it. Gobsmacked is being hit with news we're not expecting, like a life-limiting diagnosis or even a medical bill we thought our insurance would cover. We are gobsmacked.

Laws are static. Life is not. As medical conditions, care options, beliefs, attitudes, lifestyles and relationships have shifted, we've been left without the practical decision-making tools we need for self-preservation in America's complex health care game. That's reason enough to have a *Gobsmacked Preparedness Plan* at the ready. The information-gathering and decision-making tools of health literacy provide a practical and respectful means of making choices, a process rendered even more necessary with the dramatic transformations in health care access and delivery.

However, the concerns I've listed so far aren't the only challenges to health care decision making. There are other equally pressing reasons for you to be a prepared and empowered patient. As is quite often voiced in the practice of medicine, "*There may be complications* . . ." And what's coming is huge.

CHAPTER THREE

The first element of the perfect storm

By definition, a perfect storm is the collision of factors that would be manageable if each appeared separately. Together, they spell big trouble. Allow me to introduce Element Number One of the perfect storm of health care, America's demographics. You will discover that age is not the only characteristic that counts.

A pig in a python

The end of World War II meant no more sugar and gas rationing and the return of more than eleven million service personnel to peacetime life.[38] What happened in the 18 years following the celebratory date of September 2, 1945 was a demographic phenomenon never experienced before or since in the United States. There were 2.9 million babies born in 1945, which was 81,000 less than the previous year. Then the war ended, the troops came home and annual births jumped by 553,000 in 1946. The next year, the number rose to 3.8 million and so it went, until more than four million babies had been born every single year for over a decade, from 1954 through 1964.[39]

There's a plethora of theories about what really caused this boom. They cover all the bases: relative income, marital fertility, good household appliances, bad contraceptive appliances, women pushed out of war-time work and newly-created tax exemptions. Regardless, this baby-palooza was exceptional in its sudden and dramatic increase in numbers, besides its tenure. By 1964, 75.9 million babies had been born in the United States, making the Boomer cohort larger than each of its predecessors, The Greatest Generation and The Silent Generation. Adjusting over time for deaths, immigration and emigration, the Boomers' numbers peaked in 1999 at 78.8 million.[40]

It has been said the Boomers don't *affect* the economy—they *are* the economy. By 1964, 40 percent of the U.S. population was under age 20, and it was an opportunity to make big bucks selling anything a young person needed or just wanted. Make a ring of rigid plastic tubing, call it a hula hoop and in 1958 you could sell 25 million in a four-month period.[41] For the success of iconic brands, such as Gerber's, Mattel, Motown Records, Maybelline and Levi's, credit goes to the Boomers. How else to explain bestsellers like *Love Story*? To all the entrepreneurs who saw us coming, I say, *You're welcome.*

Small ticket items were not the only winners. From 1950 to 1970, the number of public school students grew by more than 25 million, creating a windfall for the construction industry working to get kids out of modular school classrooms. Halfway into the boom, a 1955 issue of *Architectural Forum* magazine observed, "*Every 15 minutes enough babies are born to fill another classroom and we are already 250,000 classrooms behind.*"[42] And the Boomers' economic impact didn't stop when they reached adulthood. Between the time the oldest and the youngest Boomers left the nest, home prices quadrupled.[43] We needed to fill those houses, so along came every manner of home furnishing store back when *assembly required* meant having friends over for pizza and a pony keg. When the time came for Boomers to start thinking about the kids' college and retirement, it marked the birth of the *financial planning* industry.[44] Yada yada yada. Wherever Boomers wandered, the economy followed.

In my family, we had a baby boom of our own, with five children arriving between 1946 and 1959. My mother referred to me as the *1951 model*, so I was—and continue to be—a front row witness to all things Boomer, from pogo sticks to peace sign jewelry. Which brings us to the Vietnam War. Between 1964 and 1970, 1.7 million Boomers were inducted to fight in Southeast Asia.[45] Back in 1942, Congress had lowered the minimum draft age from 21 to 18 to recruit troops needed for World War II.[46] The youth voting rights slogan, "*Old enough to fight, old enough to vote*," was resurrected by Boomers 30 years later and justifiably so. Of the 58,220 casualties in Vietnam, 60 percent were aged 21 or younger.[47] In a record-setting ratification process, the 26th Amendment to the U.S. Constitution was adopted by three fourths of the states in just over two months and signed by President Nixon on July 5, 1971. In an instant, eleven million voters were added to the electorate.[48] That's how Boomers roll: in a big way.

Leaping forward 50 years, we find Boomers now aged 57 to 75 and numbering more than 71 million. About half still aren't *seniors*, although, as you now know, 10,000 celebrate the big six-five every day. As we turn our attention to the future of health care, recognize that Boomers will not be the only ones impacted by what that future brings. If we've learned anything over the past 75 years, it's *What happens to the Boomers happens to America*. So here we go.

Hula hoops and health care

When we talk about the projected size of a demographic group, adjustments for births, deaths, immigration and emigration have been taken into account. Second, these are projections (read: educated guesses), so they're based on a lot of assumptions. As you will see in Chapter Six, assumptions can largely determine a forecast's validity. Most of us are not statisticians, so we're dependent on the competencies and inner workings at the U.S. Census Bureau, the U.S. Department of Health and Human Services and other governmental and private agencies. They've gotten very good at knowing how many people will arrive and leave, and we certainly have the capability of closely tracking Americans' health.

Keeping all that in mind, if I told you the share of the U.S. population aged 65 and older will increase 4 percent by the end of this decade, you might think, *Four percent growth? No big deal.* And you'd be right, but that's not the important statistic. You see, even though seniors' *proportion* or *share* of the U.S. population grows only 4 percent by 2030, the *number* of America's seniors will increase by *31 percent* over the same period. That means 17 million additional people aged 65 and older by the end of this decade and 30 million more by 2050.[49] Whether you call it a *Pig in a Python* or a *Silver Tsunami*, those 30 million people equate to cloning Texas and populating it entirely with oldsters. Yikes. Maybe this graphic will help:

Projections of the Older Adult Population: 2020 to 2060[50]

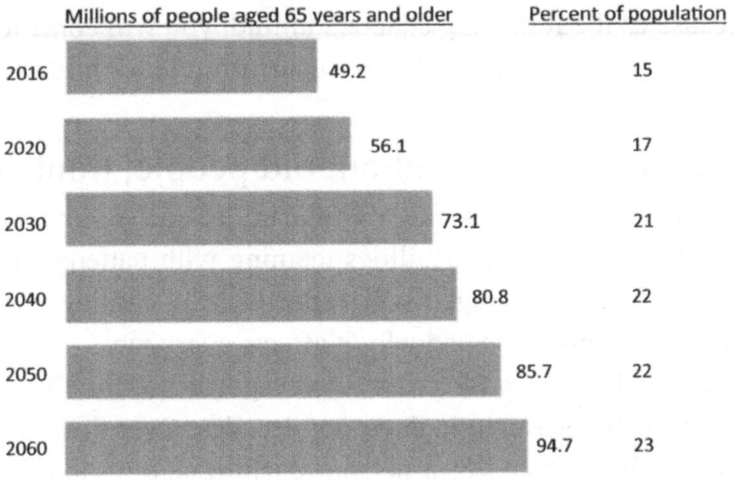

While just 4 percent growth in a cohort's share of the population may not be startling in and of itself, when you put the presence of seniors into historical perspective:

- In 1900, one in every 25 Americans was 65 or older.
- In 1994, one in every eight Americans was 65 or older.[51]
- By 2030, more than one in every five Americans will be 65 or older.

Yes, less than ten years from now, every fifth person you come across will be a senior. By any measure, that's boocoo old people. But since the Millennials now outnumber the Boomers, why still be concerned about what oldsters will need or want?

Consumers have evolving interests throughout their lives. Toddlers go for diapers and toys, teenagers like clothes and electronics and 30- and 40-somethings are focused on homes, children and vacations. Typically, demographic cohorts stay in their own lanes and don't compete for products and services. Sixty years ago, Boomers wanted hula hoops when no one else really did. Their obsession with motorcycles is over; for the most part, that's now the domain of Gen Xers and Millennials. But guess what? There's a cohort already making as many trips to the doctor as seniors. Babies. And a

40-year-old with comorbidities needs to visit as often as a 70-year-old with the same chronic conditions. With increasing frequency and intensity, the Boomers seek a cluster of services and products everyone needs to some extent: *health care*. The nature of the Boomer cohort's size, coupled with its escalating demands, are about to break all the rules. The growing presence of an older population and their mounting use of resources will shape the experience of persons of *all* ages competing with them for access to health care providers, products and services.

For more than seven decades, the Boomers have shaken America's economy, culture and politics to the core at every stage of their lives. It is foolhardy to think the health care demands of their golden years will somehow be different. Madness, really. Maybe try planning ahead for a phase in the lives of Boomers *before* it reaches crisis proportions? Because as the following chapters unfold, you will come to recognize that the Boomers are only one influence in this perfect storm of health care.

If you think this is just about old people, think again

Overcrowded classrooms sound like a headache, so just re-imagine that scenario featuring clinics, hospitals and care facilities teeming with patients. You've just seen how the population of aging and aged will expand in the coming years. Let's take a closer look at what else is going on and why it affects everyone.

Life expectancy in 1900 was 39 years. If you got a life-limiting diagnosis, your prognosis was most likely measured in days, not decades. Over time, life expectancy at birth has increased to more than 78; a person reaching age 65 today has an average remaining life of nearly 20 years.[52] Naturally, living longer increases the use of age- and health care-related resources. But to accurately estimate future needs, we have to look beyond simply the duration of life and consider a person's health status along the journey. We've seen the top illnesses that cause death: heart disease, cancer, respiratory diseases, strokes, Alzheimer's and diabetes. The good news for many is that the terminal illness of yesteryear is the lifelong manageable chronic condition of today. So a *cause of death* label and raw statistics don't begin to reflect the personal toll on a patient and loved ones who cope for years with a chronic and/or degenerative illness, not to mention the societal burdens. There's no question long disease trajectories put high demands on health care and caregiving resources. Let's take one case in point, today's sixth leading cause of death, Alzheimer's disease. It didn't even make the Top Ten until 1999. Now there are an estimated 5.8 million cases in the U.S. among those aged 65 and older, projected to be 7.1 million by 2025 and 14 million by 2050.[53] Is living with Alzheimer's the same as dying of Alzheimer's? I think not.

As for the Millennials in the audience, I'm here to say that if you believe your cohort is immune to high-maintenance and life-threatening medical issues, you have misjudged the situation. Quick review: 60 percent of *all* American adults—*everyone* aged 18 and older—have at least one chronic condition; 42 percent have two or more; and 12 percent have five or more. As a matter of fact, more than 20 million American adults have partial or complete dysfunction in at least one of these six domains: seeing, hearing, mobility, communication, cognition, or self-care—and *less than half are 65 and older.*[54] It's estimated almost half of all American adults have cardiovascular disease, with high blood pressure as the predominant diagnosis.[55] And as the prevalence of obese adults has doubled over the past 25 years, being overweight is responsible for nearly half of all chronic illness maintenance costs in America; it's estimated that 50 percent of all American adults will be medically overweight by 2030.[56]

Sorry, I'm not finished. Millennials, now aged 21 to 44, are not as healthy as the generation ahead of them. Four of the Millennials' top five chronic conditions increased in prevalence by double digits from 2014 to 2017, and one source even suggests Millennials' mortality rate could rise by more than 40 percent compared to Gen Xers.[57] We know Millennials aren't big fans of going to the doctor; more than 90 percent avoid preventive screenings and about half visit less than once a year.[58] Two things to think about, and this applies to all ages: There are many others seeking to crowd ahead of you in line, so the sooner you establish a doctor-patient relationship, the less likely you won't be able to secure one when you need one. It's not too late to take charge of one's health care—it's never too late. Second, delaying the discovery of a life-limiting disease or chronic condition often doesn't bode well. In fact, for those aged 50 and under—that's Millennials and some Gen Xers—the rate of colorectal cancer has more than doubled since the 1990s. One would expect the *number* of cases to go up as a cohort grows, but not the chances of getting a disease, especially since the overall prevalence of this cancer has declined.[59] Experts were recently prompted to lower the recommended start of colorectal cancer screenings from age 50 to age 45, even for those without exceptional risks.[60]

Moving on down the age ladder, an estimated one fourth of children under 18 now have a chronic condition. The top three chronic illnesses among children are behavioral/emotional disorders, obesity and asthma; and all have increased appreciably in recent decades.[61] In addition, one in five adolescents and one in four young adults are prediabetic.[62] All that partially explains why almost one fifth of children under age 12 take prescription medications.[63]

Regardless of your age, odds are good you or someone close to you already has one or more of these chronic conditions:

- High blood pressure
- High cholesterol
- Depression, anxiety or other mental health disorder

- Arthritis/Osteoporosis
- Chronic kidney disease
- Fibromyalgia
- Obesity
- Asthma
- Sleep apnea[64]

Although life-altering, these common ailments are not typically life-limiting, which is defined as an incurable condition ultimately shortening a person's life. They do, however, demand an abundance of medications, provider visits, emergency care, hospitalizations, therapies and lifestyle modifications.

Just more of the same old same old?

Is this pattern of chronic illness what we've seen for decades? Actually, no. Chronic conditions are now cutting even larger swaths across even more cohorts. Today's percentage of all adults with two or more chronic diseases is almost double the rate of 20 years ago.[65] Meanwhile, system-wide health care practices and policies continue to focus on acute care and curative treatments, not long-term symptom management. As consumers, we flounder, clueless on how to get specialists talking to each other, to formulate short-term treatment decisions, to access needed ancillary services and to plan for the future. Those two weakest links, communication and care coordination, add to overall systemic demands by failing to prevent disease and injury and by allowing costly and potentially harmful duplications and interactions. Then again, the prevalence of chronic illness isn't the only change afoot.

We've made turning 65 a milestone moment in America and it sort of is. Since it became the minimum age for receiving full government benefits in 1935, 65 has been tied to retirement, Social Security, getting a Medicare card and membership in a super special cohort. It's undeniable that as an earmark, being *under 65* versus being *65 and older* makes it easy to tell one herd from another. That's because each cohort's characteristics and behaviors were generally distinct from the others—and predictable. Well, things can change. Even the enduring causes of death distinguishable between age groups have undergone unexpected shifts over the past 20 years.

When we view age groups, *accidents* is the leading cause of death until age 45, it takes the third slot until age 65 and after that drops to seventh. Okay, we get it, because the behaviors of youth mean greater exposure to the risks of accidents, suicide and assault, which are the first, second and third place causes of death for those age 15 to 34. But now we're seeing an alarming rise in the *prevalence* (the *percentage* of a population with a characteristic) of fatal accidents among seniors, going from ninth to seventh place over the past two decades. In fact, *accidents* have now beaten out *influenza and pneumonia* by rank, number and rate for seniors.[66] The rate of unintentional and fatal falls for those aged 65 and older increased 31 percent from 2007 to 2016; for those aged 75 and older, it doubled from 2000 to 2016. What? More than 34,000 seniors died from unintentional falls in 2019. If the rate continues to rise, 59,000 deaths are projected for 2030.[67] These fatalities are among the three million emergency room visits, 950,000 hospitalizations and 300,000 hip fractures resulting from 35.6 million falls each year.[68]

Let's take a closer look. Again, while it's not terribly surprising there's a greater *incidence* of seniors falling because there are so many more seniors, when the *prevalence* also rises, that's worth noting. Without further research, we can only guess where the blame lies among the known risk factors for falls: chronic conditions, more frequent use of medications affecting the central nervous system and stability, blood thinners turning a bump on the head into a brain bleed, poor balance, poor nutrition and the inherent hazards that come with living longer and independently. Until we figure out the causes and act to prevent them, those who survive long enough to receive treatment will be taking places in line for emergency care, hospitalization, rehabilitation and caregiving services. So move over.

There's another piece of America's demographic puzzle that simply did not exist a few decades ago: the volume of Millennials, who outnumbered Baby Boomers as of June 2015.[69] It explains why Boomers' share of the total population isn't growing faster—they've been surpassed by the Millennials. This holds several key health care-related implications. For starters, in 2060, as the last of the Boomers wave ba-bye, the *youngest* Millennials born at the very end of the last millennium (hence the name) will be reaching their 60s. Although it's true that growth in the number of older people in America will then level off, a ginormous population of elderly will remain in place. The trend of deaths exceeding three million a year begins in 2028, numbering a quarter of a million more than in 2020. Many will be preceded by the medical complications and utilization that end of life often brings.[70] Note to Millennials: We're approaching what you will come to know as *The Wall* faster than previously thought and the issues of health care access and logistics are not going away for a very long time.

It's not even just the number of candles or diseases

Along with age and chronic illness, a person's autonomous health care needs can be linked to gender, race, ethnicity, occupation and military service. America's veterans are an example of a large cohort with health care demands unique in both nature and intensity, depending on a veteran's service experience. There is still much to learn about the progression of some service-connected diseases as our veterans age, but we already know they have a higher diagnosed prevalence of cancers, Lou Gehrig's disease (ALS), chronic obstructive pulmonary disease (COPD), diabetes, gastroesophageal reflux disease, hearing loss, substance abuse, traumatic brain injuries and post-traumatic stress disorder (PTSD).[71] Agent Orange exposure in Vietnam is linked to a higher incidence of leukemia, Hodgkin's disease, ischemic heart disease, multiple myeloma, Parkinson's disease, non-Hodgkin's lymphoma, cancers, hypothyroidism and respiratory ailments, among others.[72] The Hepatitis C infection rate for Boomer veterans is five times that of other veterans (true of *all* Boomers compared to nonBoomers),[73] more than one fourth of veterans have service-connected disabilities[74] and the suicide rate for veterans is 50 percent higher than for adult nonveterans.[75]

Shameful, but there has not been a full and detailed accounting of the United States veteran population since the nationwide census of 2000.[76] As of 2018, there were about six million living Vietnam veterans, but, as stated in the Institute of Medicine's (IOM) 2018 report, *Veterans and Agent Orange*, data on veterans' deaths relating to Agent Orange exposure "*has been elusive.*" A bit of an understatement. The CDC stopped tracking Vietnam veterans' postservice deaths in 1987 and the most recent comprehensive study was done in 2000.[77] Truly shameful. We do, however, know that all living veterans have a median age of 65, and that only half are now enrolled in the Veterans Health Administration (VHA).[78] Even though the total veteran population is projected to decline 9 percent by 2030, the number of veterans enrolled in and using the VHA has gone up 70 percent over the past 20 years, and nearly half of enrollees are aged 65 and older. Utilization of veterans' health care resources in the coming years will depend on eligibility criteria and the United States' involvement in conflicts, as well as the increasing prevalence of health conditions among aging veterans. Still, it's a good bet demand won't be going down in the foreseeable future.

It looks like Baby Boomers aren't quite done influencing America's culture and economy. If all that makes you want to grab a lawn chair and get an early spot in line, then you appreciate how utilization of and competition for health care are both on the rise. You're somewhere on the health care spectrum: young and healthy, living with a life-limiting diagnosis, managing a chronic illness or simply aging into the natural progression of increased medical and caregiving needs. In any case, you will have stiff competition to see a doctor, get emergency care, have a medical test, fill a prescription, access caregiving and use a variety of therapies. Now is the time to appreciate that just because we've assembled an amazing array of health care resources in America is no guarantee everyone will have full and unfettered access to them. Failing to be mindful of what's happening and to make necessary preparations may cost you in both quality and quantity of life. Clearly, Boomers and their elders aren't the only actors in this health care drama, but they're the undisputed headliners in the first element of health care's perfect storm, demographics. The thing is, Boomers aren't just patients . . .

CHAPTER FOUR

The second element of the perfect storm

Knowing what lies ahead allows us to make necessary plans. An abundance of people with chronic, complex and degenerative medical conditions requires substantial labor and financial resources. Will the coming years bring adequate supplies to meet these historic demands? Good question. Meet Element Number Two of the perfect storm: dwindling health care resources.

Some will pull the wagon, others will ride

As you've now seen, demographics is the first element of health care's perfect storm, dominated by cohorts of those aging and/or with chronic and complex health needs. It doesn't take a statistician to see that having a sufficient number of available workers willing and able to provide health care and caregiving is crucial to accessing those services. As we prepare to view the storm's second element, dwindling health care labor and financial resources, let's begin by looking at the *dependency ratio*, which is the relationship between the youngest or oldest in a population and those of working age (18 to 64).

Fourteen years into the baby boom, 1960, the *youth dependency ratio* was at a high of 65: there were 65 children under age 18 for every 100 people aged 18 to 64. At the same time, the *old age dependency ratio* was 17 people aged 65 and older for every 100 workers. Together, they gave us a *total dependency ratio* of 82 in the 1960s (the young and old who were dependent on those neither young nor old) and it's still a record.[79] As Boomers aged into adulthood, the youth dependency ratio fell and now remains steadily in the high 30s (30 kids versus 100 workers). Meanwhile, the old age dependency ratio has risen 40 percent since 2000 and is projected to increase another 25 percent by the end of this decade. In 2000, it translated to five working-age people for every senior; by 2030, there will be less than three,[80] pushing the *total* dependency ratio back up to 75 by 2034. That's when we'll reach another demographic milestone: For the first time in United States history, America's oldsters will outnumber its youngsters.[81]

Eenie meenie chili beanie, the spirits are about to speak

No need for a crystal ball because there are time-honored methods for making *estimates* of our present population and *projections* of future demographic trends. The Census Bureau has been doing it for eons, based on the results of each official decennial census and the American Community Surveys conducted in between. Census Bureau projections rely on statistical samplings of those who answer their surveys, as we were all encouraged to do in 2020. Incorporating factors such as fertility and mortality rates and net migration into those figures, the Census Bureau then estimates and projects the size, age, gender, ethnicity, living arrangements and even health characteristics of the population and its various cohorts.

In a similar way, we should be able to forecast the health care system's readiness to meet its future labor demands. Those projections would incorporate present workforce supply/demand numbers; utilization rates; health care provider-to-population ratios; anticipated advances in technology, services and products; workers coming into and leaving the health care profession; and the profile of Future Patient. The nature and accuracy of applied assumptions determine the credibility and trustworthiness of the resulting projections, which are then relied on by policy makers, stakeholders, educators—and now you and me.

The statistical why and wherefore of projections is way above my pay scale as a statistician, since I am not one. For our purposes, let's you and I think in terms of simpler, perhaps even logical, queries such as:

- *How many health care workers are there?*
- *Is the need for health care workers currently being met?*
- *How many health care workers will we need?*
- *What goes into making a reliable projection?*
- *Will there be a shortage or a surplus?*

How many health care workers are there?

This just might knock your socks off. An estimated 15 million people work in America's health care industry. As an occupational category, *health care* has 76 distinct careers within it,[82] and that's just a start. For instance, among the one million physicians and surgeons licensed in the United States are 120 different types of specialists and subspecialists.[83] Within the 700,000 to 900,000 active practitioners,[84] about one third are primary care physicians, i.e., family care doctors, internists, pediatricians, geriatricians and gynecologists.[85]

As for registered nurses, there are between three and four million licensees, with about three million actively employed.[86] The largest category of health care labor, *direct care workers,* are those responsible for your hands-on care while hospitalized, receiving at-home assistance, in rehab or at a nursing facility. They include home health aides, personal care aides, nursing assistants and orderlies, and they number about five million.[87] Oh, and those 15 million health care workers do *not* include those in related fields, such as health care facility construction and management, information technology, biomedical engineering and health insurance.

Here are current workforce estimates for a few of the health care professionals we rely upon, besides physicians and registered nurses:

- Dentists – 151,600
- Direct care workers – 5,018,800
- Licensed practical and vocational nurses – 721,700
- Nurse practitioners – 211,300
- Pharmacists – 321,700
- Physical therapists – 258,200
- Physician assistants – 125,500
- Psychiatrists – 27,900
- Social workers in health care, mental health and substance abuse – 308,200[88]

Is the need for health care workers currently being met?

Good question. Other than anecdotal evidence from those who struggle to fill positions,[89] there's not a lot of empirical data. Here's what we do know. The health care sector accounts for 11 percent of all employment in the United States. Its growth has been nearly three times that of other industries since the last recession began in 2007.[90] And despite the layoffs resulting from COVID-19, this job sector is still expanding; as of September 2020, the number of health care jobs was only 4.2 percent below prepandemic numbers.[91] We're just beginning to appreciate how many health care professionals are choosing to take early retirement or seek alternative positions rather than return after pandemic furloughs, but we know there was already a problem filling those jobs before March 2020. It now seems much worse. How does all this impact projections for satisfying future health care labor needs? We're still unsure, except we know this sector sustains more than 900,000 businesses, 20 million employees and one trillion dollars in annual payroll,[92] and *Health Care and Social Assistance* was among eight industry categories experiencing historic *job opening highs* in 2019. There were 1.3 million unfilled positions in health care and social assistance before the pandemic struck.[93]

Sorry, but I find nothing on current supply versus demand for physicians. For the overall nursing industry, job vacancies stand at 8 percent, with over half of hospitals reporting 7.5 percent of jobs open; that's more than a 10 percent increase since 2015. Just consider the disruption in job performance if the average turnover rate is 94 percent—more than nine of every ten nurses are replaced each year.[94] In 2018, the Veterans Health Administration reported 40,456 vacancies, which means 11 percent of its jobs were unfilled.[95] As for direct care workers, there's no hard data on job openings, but 2009's turnover rate of 39 percent rose to 82 percent by 2018. Needing to replace more than eight workers of every ten in a year's time causes more than half of surveyed agencies to turn clients away.[96]

The primary source of current health care labor data research is, or should be, the Health Resources and Services Administration (HRSA), an agency within the US. Department of Health and Human Services (HHS). One reason it's responsible for tracking labor data in health care professions is to identify *Health Professional Shortage Areas* (HPSAs) across the country. HRSA sets the minimum population-to-primary care provider (PCP) ratio at 3,500-to-one to avoid an HPSA designation. And their conclusion? The number of HPSAs for PCPs throughout the country has more than doubled since 2003,[97] we have less than half the PCPs we currently need and it would take 15,575 additional PCPs to fill that gap. These HPSAs represent over 83 million in population.[98] Similarly, less than 30 percent of minimum staffing for dentists is being met; we could use 10,919 more right now. According to the HRSA, psychiatrists are at only 27 percent of the recommended supply and it would take 6,398 more to correct the existing shortage.[99] (Funny story. In Chapter Six I'll share how the federal government finally noticed it's been mistakenly including 46,000 hospitalists in the census of available primary care providers. Oops.)

Having a benchmark of one primary care physician for 3,500 in population might make you wonder: *What is a reasonable number of patients for a doctor to serve?* We measure that by *patient panel size*, which is the number of persons under a physician's care over the prior 12 to 18 months. For example, a provider who works 240 days a year seeing a patient every 20 minutes could have a patient panel of 2,072, based on an average 2.78 visits per year per patient.[100] Many variables shape an optimal panel size: the ages and general health of the patients; the provider's practice style; the location's population density; whether a health care team is in place; and the use of technology, such as medical scribes, voice recognition software and telemedicine. Studies show panel sizes actually range from 983 to 2,600 patients. A panel of 2,600 patients translates to an average of 30 patients seen for 18 minutes each in a nine-hour day (sorry, no breaks for lunch or even coffee and no transition time between appointments).

The long-held industry standard of 2,500-patient panels is based on 15 to 20-year-old demographic data not reflective of the modern demands of aging and chronically ill patients. It also predates the electronic health record burden providers now bear, which requires data input during each patient visit, as well as computer time outside direct care hours.[101] Nurses and doctors spend one fourth to one half of their time each day on a tablet or personal computer, updating patient charts and inputting administrative and regulatory information.[102] Couple all that with consistent research showing a doctor's average caseload is only 20 patients per day—not 30. Even that load requires a 51-hour work week and reflects a patient panel of only 1,726 patients, which is less than half the ratio used for HPSA estimates of underserved populations across the country.

What will continue to come from even more high-maintenance patients and the heightened demands of technology? Eighty-one percent of surveyed physicians say their practices are at capacity or already overextended.[103] Other research shows it takes an average of 29 days to see a new family physician in a large metro market (high of 109 days in Boston); and 56 days for mid-sized markets (Yakima, Washington took the prize at 153 days). From 2014 to 2017, the average wait time rose 30 percent for all specialties in large metro markets.[104] Compare your own experience in accessing a physician. Your zip code may be the problem.

Our dependence on anecdotal evidence rather than hard data raises more questions:

- *Are HPSA population-to-provider ratios based on the real world of health care?* That's difficult to believe unless we assume either half the patients will never actually visit the doctor, or doctors are willing and able to work more than 100 hours a week. Consider the illustrative case of hospice and palliative care physicians in Anchorage, Alaska versus St. Paul, Minnesota. The two groups merit nearly identical physician-to-population ratios. The reality is St. Paul has 34 of these comfort care specialists, who are aided by 56 more in adjacent Minneapolis. In stark contrast, their 16 counterparts in Anchorage must cross 663,000 square miles to reach patients.[105]
- *What if a patient panel doesn't reflect the nation's overall demographics?* Those under one year of age see the doctor more than two and a half times the average of 2.78 visits, while those over age 64 are at almost twice the average.[106] So, how many babies and seniors are in the provider's panel? Is the doctor in an urban or rural setting? Both impact accessibility, and older residents' share of rural populations has grown 60 percent over the past four decades.[107]
- *Does panel size vary with the provider's medical specialty?* The frequency of a patient's visits often matches the trajectory of a chronic condition. It may mean more work for specialists, but it can also mean a greater burden on primary care physicians who continue to manage a patient's disease because there is simply no specialist close by. In intense treatment protocols, such as palliative and hospice care, it's been suggested that seeing eight patients a day is more realistic than 30.[108]

When it comes to available and reliable data on the existing health care workforce, we'll have to go with what we have, rather than what we wish for.

How many health care workers will we need?

Previewing future health care labor needs takes us one step closer to the ultimate analysis of whether there will be a surplus or a deficit. How will that impact your access to a neurologist if you're having a stroke? Or the ability to get a mammogram soon after finding a lump in your breast? Or the freedom to transport your loved one from the hospital directly to a hospice for crucial palliative care?

Might as well swallow the biggest pills first: Although the rate of population growth is slowing, the Census Bureau projects the United States will nevertheless have a net gain of between 21 and 22 million residents by 2030, bringing our population to 355 million.[109] Gains in employment across all U.S. industry sectors will slow, adding six million jobs from 2019 to 2029. There is, however, one industry projected to grow by 15 percent—four times the national average—and it accounts for more than half of those six million new jobs: *Health care and social assistance.*[110]

If you were considering a career as a wind turbine service technician, good thinking. It's first in the list of fastest growing occupations between now and 2029, according to the U.S. Department of Labor's Bureau of Labor Statistics (BLS). The rest look like a health care job fair, with half of the nation's 30 fastest growing occupations coming from the medical arena and adding more than three million jobs from 2019 to 2029.[111] These projections from the BLS take into account broad social and demographic trends and the general economy. However, because they focus on the *labor* side rather than the *consumer* side of the ledger, BLS projections may or may not reflect all the health care-related issues we covered in Chapter Three, such as aging, chronic illness, lifestyle choices and medical advances.[112]

Before I share specifics about those three million new health care jobs, it's important to understand BLS projections are of employment and occupational trends only. Whether there will be workers available to fill the demands of projected job growth is another matter entirely. A good example is direct care workers. The BLS projects this sector will have nearly 1.3 million *additional* jobs by 2029, but that doesn't take into account the estimated 6.9 million openings resulting from employees' job changes or retirements.[113] The BLS model also assumes supply equals demand throughout the projection period, even if that doesn't reflect reality.

<u>Occupation</u> / **<u>Projected job growth from 2019 to 2029</u>** / <u>Rate of growth</u>

Dentists / **+4,000** / 3%

Direct care workers / **+1,279,000** / 26%

Licensed practical/vocational nurses / **+65,700** / 9%

Nurse practitioners / **+110,700** / 52%

Pharmacists / **-10,500** / -3%

Physical therapists / **+47,000** / 18%

Physician assistants / **+39,300** / 31%

Physicians and surgeons / **+24,000** / 4%

Psychiatrists / **+3,300** / 12%

Registered nurses / **+221,900** / 7%

Social workers in health care/mental health/substance abuse / **+47,400** / 16%

You've already learned enough about health care's perfect storm to not be surprised, right? Well, maybe that one standout, pharmacists. The BLS attributes this reduction in jobs to greater use of mail order versus retail prescriptions, along with more reliance on pharmacy technicians, an occupation projected to gain 15,200 positions.[114]

Since our population is growing both in age and in the incidence of chronic illness, it's not unreasonable to find the demand for health care services, products and personnel going *up*—not *down*—over the coming years. Here's a brief review of why:

- While the total U.S. population grows only 7 percent by 2030, the number of seniors increases by 31 percent, leaving us with 17 million more than today.
- Seventy-five percent of America's seniors and 42 percent of all adults have two or more chronic conditions.
- An estimated 48 percent of American adults have cardiovascular disease.
- The prevalence of obese adults has nearly doubled over the past 25 years and is projected to represent half of all American adults by 2030.
- For Millennials, the incidence of four of their top five chronic conditions increased by double digits from 2014 to 2017.
- One fourth of children under age 18 have a chronic medical condition, and 20 percent of those under age 12 are taking prescription medications.

Within that gain of 22 million people by 2030, growth in the number of seniors will be ten times that of minors.[115] That matters because as a population ages and has more chronic conditions, health care labor needs increase, as we have already witnessed:

- Aging impedes mobility and independence and—surprise—the need for direct care workers increased 55 percent from 2008 to 2018.[116]
- The number of emergency department visits for those aged 45 to 64 rose 20 percent from 2005 to 2016.
- More than half of seniors' physician appointments are prompted by a chronic condition; they make 48 percent more trips to the emergency department than young people and are admitted to the hospital more than one third of the time.[117]
- For *all* Americans over the age of 17, a chronic condition is the most common reason to see a doctor.[118]

In making educated guesses about future labor demands, the demographics of aging and chronic illness are not the only variables to consider. The Association of American Medical Colleges has identified other equally daunting prospects:

- If folks made healthier lifestyle choices and improved their health outcomes, we'd need 33,900 more doctors than already projected to cover the years of increased longevity. Sometimes you just can't win.
- When doctors work even 2 to 3 percent fewer hours per week, which they've been doing over the past couple of years, it equates to losing the services of 19,200 full-time physicians. Based on a 2,000-patient panel, that leaves 38 million patients without providers. When dealing in health care, think *volume.*[119]
- If we figured out how to better serve those with inadequate—or no—access to health care, most probably the current need for providers would increase by anywhere from 74,100 to 180,000 doctors. Careful what we promise.

To those uncertainties I would add these unknowables in estimating future health care labor needs:

- Fluctuating economic conditions and how they impact education, hiring and retirement decisions, on both employer and employee sides of the table.
- Health care reform of any kind that affects health care access and utilization and how it is paid for.
- Stakeholders' and policyholders' acknowledgement of the strains on financial and human resources and any efforts they make to implement remedial plans.
- The extent of providers' burnout and their willingness to tough it out until they reach 65, which is the assumed retirement age in most projections.
- And I can hardly believe I'm writing this—our response to the next pandemic.

As Ed Sullivan used to say: "*Dude, that's a lot of plates in the air.*" Well, maybe he didn't say it, but I'll bet he was thinking it.

What goes into making a reliable projection?

We're getting closer to the educated guesses. Before we view the expert schmexperts' opinions, there are some forecasting basics and limitations to keep in mind:

- *How many health care workers are there now and is the need currently being met?* It's standard practice to assume supply equals demand at the beginning of a projection period, even if it flies in the face of the most recent job surveys, designated Health Professional Shortage Areas and reports from the health care recruiting industry.

- *How many health care workers will we need in the future?* The growth of the U.S. population and the increasing number of those aging and/or chronically ill can be easily estimated. Both groups are more frequent users of health care resources and we've already seen the trending prevalence. In light of America's demographics, it seems counterintuitive to assume current levels of health care utilization and staffing will remain unchanged, but that is the prevailing assumption.

- *How many people will leave and enter the health care profession?* Reliable estimates of losses and gains come from statistics on deaths, retirements, job changes and new hires. More than half of surveyed physicians plan to retire within five years[120] (a little disconcerting, since only one third were 60 years old when asked). Still, even assuming retirement does not occur until age 65, one fourth of *all* current health care workers qualify by 2030, and *half* reach retirement age by 2035. Among specialties, such as pulmonology, psychiatry, cardiology and rheumatology, the percentages are even higher.[121] (More about how physicians are responding to burnout in Chapter Eight.)

Similarly, about half of nurses are aged 50 and older, one third will reach retirement age between 2023 and 2028 and an estimated one million will leave the health care industry throughout this decade.[122] Failing to acknowledge the irreplaceable know-how and mentoring that departs with them is naïve and hazardous to our health. An estimated 1.7 million years of nursing experience vanished in 2015 alone, double what we lost in 2005.[123] Much like the aging demographics of doctors and nurses, 30 percent of home health care workers (part of the direct care workforce) are aged 55 and older.[124]

And the number of health care professionals entering the field? About 26,000 doctors now graduate from medical school each year, which reflects a 35 percent increase from 2008 to 2019.[125] The annual number of new medical licensees rose 21 percent from 2010 to 2018, when it reached 32,601.[126] All good news, although for more than 23 years there was an unresolved issue over the lack of funding for residencies (more about that in Chapter Six). One hundred fifty thousand registered nurses receive a degree and become licensed each year,[127] as we turn away an estimated 75,000 qualified applicants, largely due to a lack of nursing faculty.[128]

With rare exceptions for forecasts that address the issue of underserved populations in their narratives, the workforce projections following here are based on consumers' historical *demand* for health care services only, which is not the same as *need. Need* is the level of health care people would seek and receive if they were fully informed and responsible concerning their health care (read: health literate) *and* they had unfettered access to resources. Available projections address only what consumers will ask for in the future based on the past, not necessarily what they really need or would seek if they could. Meeting the currently underserved physical and mental health care needs of our population is *not* baked into the assumptions. In fact, it would be catastrophically overwhelming for the health care system to even attempt that. For example, in its projections for psychiatrists, HHS notes mental health care in 2013 was accessed by only 45 percent of Americans estimated to have mental illness, leaving a possible 40 to 45 million individuals needing help but not receiving it.[129]

Last, but not least, projections not only attempt to forecast the behavior of humans, they are also the work of humans, with all their unique perspectives and biases. Keep that in mind as you witness how all this data shakes out in the hands of professional prognosticators.

So? Will there be a shortage or a surplus?

It's obvious the availability of an adequate and competent health care workforce directly impacts our ability to access health care, which is why having reliable and up-to-date projections is crucial to planning, on both systems and individual levels. In Chapter Six, you'll have the opportunity to look back a few decades and witness just how profoundly workforce projections influence policy and, consequently, touch our lives in very personal ways. Once you see what today's policy makers and stakeholders are relying upon, it may appear projections are more art than science. Perhaps even more science fiction than art.

This is a comprehensive review of the projections of future physician **shortages**:

Date	Source	When	Projected shortage
2015	AAMC	2025	46,000 – 90,000 physicians[130]
2016	AAMC	2025	61,700 – 94,700 physicians[131]
2017	AAMC	2030	40,800 – 104,900 physicians[132]
2018	AAMC	2030	42,600 – 121,300 physicians[133]
2018	MHPA	2025	11,000 physicians[134]
2019	AAMC	2032	46,900 – 121,900 physicians[135]
2020	Zhang	2025	72,472 physicians
2020	Zhang	2030	139,160 physicians[136]
2020	AAMC	2033	54,100 – 139,000 physicians
2021	AAMC	2034	37,800 – 124,000 physicians[137]

These are **shortages** projected for registered nurses:

Date	Source	When	Projected shortage
2012	Juraschek	2030	918,232 registered nurses[138]
2018	Zhang	2025	336,336 registered nurses
2018	Zhang	2030	510,394 registered nurses[139]

Zeroing in on some specialties and health care support occupations, these projected **shortages** are not any more optimistic:

Date	Source	When	Projected shortage
2015	HRSA	2025	15,600 dentists[140]
2015	Lin	2030	195,850 social workers[141]

2016	HRSA	2025	23,640 primary care physicians[142]
2016	HRSA	2025	26,670 – 250,510 mental health professionals[143]
2017	HRSA	2025	26,980 geriatricians[144]
2018	MHPA	2025	541,300 direct care workers
2018	MHPA	2025	58,700 medical/clinical lab technologists
2018	MHPA	2025	40,000 medical/lab technicians
2018	MHPA	2025	29,400 nurse practitioners[145]
2018	Lupu	2040	2,540-5,000 hospice/PC doctors[146]
2019	HRSA	2030	17,990 – 21,150 adult psychiatrists[147]
2019	AAMC	2032	21,100 – 55,200 primary care physicians
2020	AAMC	2033	21,400 – 55,200 primary care physicians
2021	AAMC	2034	17,800 – 48,000 primary care physicians[148]
2020	HRSA	2030	12,530 adult psychiatrists
2020	HRSA	2030	11,530 addiction counselors[149]

Now, here are projected **surpluses** in health care labor, all from the HHS subagency, the Health Resources and Services Administration (HRSA). Just to be clear, these projections all forecast the number of health care-related workers who should plan on being *unemployed* in the coming years because we will not be needing their services:

Date	**Source**	**When**	**Projected surplus**
2014	HRSA	2025	340,000 registered nurses[150]
2017	HRSA	2030	293,800 registered nurses[151]
2018	HRSA	2030	18,640 – 50,720 pharmacists[152]
2018	HRSA	2030	23,550 – 23,960 occupational therapists
2018	HRSA	2030	3,540 – 7,100 physical therapists[153]
2019	HRSA	2030	200,280 – 253,660 social workers[154]
2019	HRSA	2030	3,720 – 4,310 juvenile psychiatrists[155]
2020	HRSA	2030	244,620 social workers
2020	HRSA	2030	640 juvenile psychiatrists[156]
2020	HRSA	2030	1,080 dentists[157]

(Yeah, well, if you think your head hurts, imagine how mine feels.) Admittedly, what I don't know about the behind-the-curtain algorithms and analyses of workforce supply and demand projections is a lot. But I think I speak for all of us when I say, "*I do not have a better idea of future health care access for having seen these forecasts*." Maybe you're as puzzled as I: *When two projections are dramatically different, isn't at least one of them wrong?*

How about the conspicuous absence of any HHS/HRSA projections for physicians? That's because HHS has not produced data on the existing census of all doctors since

2001 and has never provided supply/demand projections for the physician workforce beyond 2020. True story. A classic policy of *Don't ask/Don't have to answer*. It escapes me why educational institutions, big providers, payers and groups claiming to advocate for America's aging and most vulnerable residents are not throwing a major hissy over this. On what are they basing their own strategic plans? Do they have strategic plans?

Forget about them. What about you and me? As patients and advocates trying to make informed preparations for self-care, like those you'll learn about in Chapters Eleven through Sixteen, we could use some reliable information. Hey, we just want to know whether there will be an unmet demand for health care resources and whether it will cut into our access. We know from personal observations that no one element of health care stands alone; the moving parts rely on each other for the best health outcomes. Will I lose independence because I can't access timely physical therapy? Is the emergency doctor diagnosing my chest pains the only one who applied for the job? How long will I have to wait for test results when there's no radiologist available? For us, these are the pertinent questions that remain unanswered by these irreconcilable—and in some cases, indefensibly outdated and bizarre—projections. If there exist credible, comprehensive, consistent and conclusive answers to the question, *Are we facing a shortage or a surplus of health care workers?*, I'm not seeing them.

When all else fails, resort to logic

Let's focus on information you and I already have and use it to reflect on the projections from HRSA and others. Then let's make some logical and useful forecasts of our own. What do we know so far? Well, we have solid data showing:

- ✓ Chronic conditions, aging and population growth are inflating the rate of health care utilization.
- ✓ The health care industry will grow by three million jobs over the next ten years.
- ✓ Changing work patterns and aging employees are shrinking the number of available health care workers to perform those duties.
- ✓ Many areas of health care already have unfillable job openings.
- ✓ We're not licensing as many doctors and nurses as we could be.

I'm also not a physicist, but even I understand there are still only 24 hours in a day. In what universe does all we know about demographics and demand (current and future) add up to a projected surplus in *any* health care occupation? Seriously, what is the deal with the dueling analyses of the nursing workforce, made just a year apart yet separated by 800,000 workers? Or the science behind forecasts of either a 195,000 shortfall or a 250,000 surplus among social workers? Or the reasoning that supports a projection of

4,310 *excess* juvenile psychiatrists when HPSA data shows slightly over one fourth of mental health needs currently being met?

The suicide rate for those aged 10 to 24 increased over 50 percent from 2007 to 2018, and suicide remains the second leading cause of death for those aged 14 to 18.[158] Recall that HRSA previously acknowledged 40 to 45 million persons with mental health needs (adults *and* juveniles) are being grossly underserved. Now we're to accept the assertion in HRSA's 2019 projection that the HPSA gap will be filled by 2030 and still leave thousands of unemployable juvenile psychiatrists hanging about.[159] Alternatively, we can look to the 2020 projection for 2030 in which there is only a 640 juvenile psychiatrist surplus. Of course, the assumptions for that particular forecast do not in any way address inadequacies or existing mental health worker shortages. Do we take that to mean HHS simply no longer plans to provide mental health services for individuals presently underserved?

In truth, thinking people would never imagine it's even possible to have too many mental health professionals—ever. This makes one wonder which of these conflicting and preposterous HHS projections, if any, are being relied upon by policy makers and stakeholders as they prioritize health care spending. You know, this makes one wonder about many things.

When somebody says it's not about the money . . .

. . . it's about the money.[160] We've covered health care labor, but the perfect storm's second element also encompasses declining *financial* resources. Although prioritizing health care spending is the domain of policy makers and stakeholders, the trickle-down consequences of their decisions are potentially life-altering for health care consumers. As patients and advocates, there are inherent risks in having someone else decide whether you need and deserve recommended medical care.

It might be helpful at this point to grasp what it really means when we talk about *a trillion dollars*. If I hand you one dollar bill every second, I'll make you a millionaire in 12 days. At the same rate, guess how long it takes to become a *trillionaire.* Just shy of 32,000 years. Do the math. Keep that in mind as you hear the term *trillion* so blithely tossed around by those who control the spending of it.

Total health care costs in the United States were $3.8 trillion in 2019, and are projected to reach $6.2 trillion by 2028, with nearly half being financed by local, state and federal governments. Health care spending's share of the Gross Domestic Product has more than doubled since 1970 and is now at 17.7 percent.[161] And annual costs per person, now at $11,582, have increased 150 percent over the past two decades.[162] Quelle surprise, but demographics explain much of this growth. Until age 44, Americans are a bargain, as their share of health care spending is far less than their portion of the population. Middle-aged Americans, aged 45 to 54, are even stephen: they account for 13 percent of both the population and health care spending. Then we come to those I will simply refer to as the *Boomers+ Gang,* Americans aged 57 and older. They comprise 29 percent of the population, but claim 56 percent of the health care spending.[163] There's the rub: Because we've done such a good job of extending lives, it's estimated by 2030 we'll have 8.6 years of disability at life's end—1.2 years more than in 2010.[164] There's a cost for keeping people alive longer.

Chronic medical conditions are a huge driver of health care expenses. More than one third of that $3.8 trillion in spending is for the direct care of chronic illnesses (in-patient, out-patient, and medications), with more than half of the Medicare budget spent on just 17 percent of its beneficiaries, the ones having six or more chronic conditions. Sixty percent of the population aged two and older are either obese or overweight (and that's prepandemic); obesity-related conditions account for $1.7 trillion in health care spending. These staggering numbers are the annual direct health costs and indirect lost economic productivity costs of leading chronic diseases for patients of all ages:

- Alzheimer's Disease - $268,300,000,000
- Cancers - $281,000,000,000
- Diabetes - $526,600,000,000
- Arthritis and Back Pain - $843,400,000,000
- Cardiovascular Conditions - $1,461,300,000,000[165]

For many chronic illnesses, caregiving needs are not far behind demands for direct medical care. One in three people requires either temporary or long-term residential skilled nursing care at some point and Medicaid foots the bill for 60 percent of them.[166] More than 25 percent of Medicare patients with Alzheimer's rely on Medicaid for their residential care, as compared to only 11 percent of other Medicare beneficiaries. It's little wonder: the total lifetime cost of caring for an Alzheimer's patient is an estimated $357,000,[167] which further illustrates the distinction between *dying of* Alzheimer's and *living with* Alzheimer's. And that only takes into account those who have paid care. Many millions of others rely on an army of uncompensated caregivers who provide 83 percent of all assistance given to frail and elderly persons, help that is otherwise unavailable due to a lack of both funds and workers. In fact, an estimated 53 million people, over one fifth of U.S. adults, now act as unpaid caregivers for a child or adult with special needs, up nearly 10 million caregivers since 2015. A fourth of them are caring for two or more others. Their time equates to 65 billion hours of labor provided gratis every year, which is an estimated savings of $1.6 trillion in annual health care costs.[168] There are no public or private funds available to replace this generosity of spirit, assuming we could find persons willing and able to do the work, which we cannot. And those 35.6 million accidental falls now occurring each year? They account for $50 billion of health care spending.[169] Remember, think *volume*.

Whatever you do, don't make eye contact

Yes, there's a 700-pound gorilla in the corner. Medicare is the largest single purchaser of personal health care, with an annual budget of $800 billion that accounts for more than one fifth of all health care spending. A government-issued health insurance policy for those aged 65 and older and some disabled persons, Medicare spending is due to reach $1 trillion by 2022 and grow 7.6 percent every year until 2028. Seventy-seven percent of Medicare spending is for seniors (excluding those with end-stage renal disease). Nineteen percent is for those receiving Medicare as part of Social Security Disability Insurance.[170] In 2010, average lifetime Medicare benefits paid were $131,000; by 2030, it's expected to be closer to $223,000. Medicare's counterpart, Medicaid, insures beneficiaries who have lower incomes and/or are disabled and its annual budget of $614 billion is not far behind Medicare's.[171]

This is another case of demographic's one-two punch. The money that funds Medicare comes from payroll taxes, the premiums paid by beneficiaries and general revenue dollars authorized by Congress. (That last category has been the largest source of Medicare funding since 2009.) Medicare Part A is paid for through payroll taxes and has been heading for a fiscal brick wall since 2008. Not surprising, since the workers-to-beneficiary ratio was 4.6 when the program began and is now 2.9; it's projected to be 2.5 by 2028. The Medicare HI Trust Fund that helps pay for Part A could be exhausted as early as 2023. So there you go. Like a household with a solvency issue, there are two choices: bring in more money or spend less. Indeed, the Medicare Payment Advisory Commission (MedPAC) has suggested raising payroll taxes by 31 percent or reducing Part A spending by 19 percent.[172] Either potential solution is going to be bad news for someone.

Rural hospitals also illustrate how an aging population reduces revenue while raising costs. Their communities tend to have older residents, with lower incomes and more chronic conditions. As a result, rural facilities have greater dependence on government-funded health care than their urban counterparts. Medicare and Medicaid patients cause a heavier paperwork burden, even as their lower reimbursement schedules impact the hospital's ability to acquire the latest equipment and attract and retain health care professionals.[173] One hundred thirty rural hospitals have already closed over the past decade,[174] which is a serious issue if you're the patient who must access preventive, chronic, acute and emergency care from a life-threatening distance. In fact, more than half the counties in the United States don't have one single intensive care bed, an issue-turned-lethal-circumstance during the COVID-19 crisis.[175] Geographically challenged.

For the record, Medicare is not a free ride for recipients. A monthly premium is paid by most, along with the cost of supplemental insurance (MSI) for the 20 percent of costs not covered by Medicare; that ranges from $67 to $481 per month. (The managed care model known as Medicare Advantage, offered at little or no cost to enrollees, eliminates the need for MSI and is used by one third of Medicare beneficiaries.) With premiums, co-pays, deductibles and noncovered items, the average Medicare enrollee spent $5,460 for health care in 2016. Those with a chronic condition can expect to pay from $10,000 to $12,000 in out-of-pocket expenses per year.[176] To put this into perspective, average Medicare out-of-pocket spending in 2013 was 41 percent of an individual's Social Security benefit. It's projected to be 50 percent by 2030.[177] Nearly half of those surveyed say they already have difficulty affording health care. Is it any surprise half to two thirds of Americans are concerned about health care costs? Equally disturbing is that patients often feel compelled to solve that financial challenge by not seeking medical care when needed.[178]

In the private sector, commercial health insurers' $1.2 trillion in annual spending accounts for 31 percent of national health care costs, about $6,000 per person. Employers spend over $7,000 for single employee coverage and more than $21,000 for a family policy, 55 percent more than ten years ago. Annual out-of-pocket spending for health care is $407 billion,[179] which includes about $7,000 per family for premium contributions and/or medical co-pays.[180] It all adds up quickly.

This chapter focused on whether the demographics of both patients and providers will cause an imbalance in meeting the health care workforce demands of the coming years. In spite of policy makers' failure to provide up-to-date, reliable or plausible guidance, you and I have enough compelling evidence to draw our own conclusions. It is not looking good. Furthermore, as the health care workforce shrinks, finances are squeezed by dwindling revenue and increased costs. We are about to see how a lack of health literacy will join the first two elements of health care's perfect storm to produce a trifecta—and this is not a winning combination.

CHAPTER FIVE

The third element of the perfect storm

When you're sitting in an overcrowded clinic waiting to be seen by an overworked doctor, you better bring your medical decision making A Game. Navigating the health care system without the skills to preserve patient rights to informed consent, autonomy and safety is dangerous. It's also Element Number Three of the perfect storm: the lack of health literacy.

I'm putting on my advocacy hat and standing up for *health literacy*, a much maligned and misconstrued notion. For starters, learning to cook vegan is not a step toward achieving health literacy. Neither are free blood pressure screenings nor salsa dancing. Yet public libraries, senior centers and health care systems across the nation promote these and similar offerings under the guise of helping their constituents become health literate. *Health literacy is recognizing when, how and where to access, process and understand basic health information and services needed to make informed medical treatment and care decisions.* Yes, being health literate may lead you to practice better eating habits, check on your blood pressure or cha-cha, but you get the point.

More of what health literacy is *not.* It is also not *functional literacy*, which is the ability to read and write. Fully comprehending information or having a translator are both good ideas, but of limited value if no one knows what questions to ask the doctor. One's level of formal education is also not a determinant of health literacy. I know some highly degreed people who don't know diddly about how to respond to an unexpected health care crisis. For some, less than diddly. With all due respect for these wise guys, they haven't a clue how to access information or effectively self advocate. Even being a medical expert may not equate to being health literate. Witness a book I highly recommend, the beautifully written *When Breath Becomes Air*, by the late Dr. Paul Kalanithi.[181] He was completing his brain surgery residency when diagnosed with advanced lung cancer. By his own admission, he had to learn how to find and evaluate treatment options as a patient in order to manage his disease and make the difficult choices facing him and his wife. This brilliant and highly-educated young brain surgeon still needed to first become a health literate patient.

Health literacy is having the needed information-gathering and decision-making skills at the ready long before you're faced with a health care challenge. It's mastering the *process* of learning, rather than the actual knowledge you will gain in applying its basics. Lacking health literacy is evocative of the expression *I don't even know what I don't know.* Once you grasp the fundamentals of being health literate, you'll recognize when to implement them and be prepared to access the information needed for shared decision making. Simply put, being health literate is having what it takes to make prudent health care decisions and never wishing you had been more empowered or engaged or informed.

Here's health literacy in action: The doctor says you have hyperlipidemia and recommends a drug regimen. Many are inclined to simply nod and say "*Okay.*" A health literate patient first asks what hyperlipidemia is. After learning it's high cholesterol, he fully explores and discusses the prognosis, treatment options, recommended lifestyle changes, potential risks and possible side effects of the disease and medications. Then—and only then—he decides whether to proceed with the new prescription. That's what shared and health literate decision making looks like.

In 2003, the U.S. Department of Education conducted a major study of Americans' ability to access and comprehend health care information needed "*to make appropriate health decisions.*" They identified the percentage of those aged 16 and older whose skills matched each level of health literacy:

- *Below basic health literacy* - 14 percent
- *Basic health literacy* - 21 percent
- *Intermediate health literacy* - 53 percent
- *Proficient health literacy* – 12 percent[182]

Those are cringeworthy findings, and if accurate, truly disturbing. Although the 2003 study was not the first to assess Americans' health literacy, it was the largest and most widely publicized at the time. Since then, a generously funded and seemingly endless effort to advance health literacy research has concluded there are virtually no signs of improvement. Thousands of studies and academic papers agree that when it comes to managing our health care, American adults are consistently and persistently inept.[183]

This lack of health literacy contributes significantly to one of the most prevalent threats to health care access, widespread chronic illness. The initial failing is in Americans' pervasive ignorance about how lifestyle choices impact health outcomes, followed by their dogged refusal to prevent and/or properly manage chronic conditions. Less than one fourth of surveyed adults realize at least 80 percent of premature chronic diseases are caused by bad healthy living choices—not bad genes.[184] In truth, the risk factors for nearly all acute and chronic killer diseases are avoidable or reversible: smoking, inactivity, lousy nutrition, obesity, excessive alcohol use, raised blood glucose and failure to get regular health screenings.[185] My intent here is not to shame, but to state a fact: The lack of health literate choices by a few—or many—will result in reduced health care access for everyone.

People with lower health literacy receive less preventive care and are hospitalized more. They are more likely to have a worse post-discharge outcome, to misuse prescriptions, to have a lower quality of life and to have a higher mortality rate—they die sooner.[186] On the other hand, those who fully understand their health care options and take every opportunity to practice shared decision making are more likely to get the treatment they prefer, receive less futile medical care and are less likely to be hospitalized at life's end.[187] Their health outcomes are optimized. A striking example are lives lost to medical errors each year, even though the fundamentals of health literacy are synonymous with steps recommended to prevent mortal mistakes.[188] Health literacy is what stands between you and being injured—or worse.

Those were illustrations of how one's level of health literacy impacts the quantity and quality of life. Then there's the money. Even before we got the results of the 2003 Department of Education study, the annual costs of low health literacy had been estimated in the tens of billions of dollars. And that was over 20 years ago. Expenses directly related to the improper and unnecessary use of medications each year alone are estimated at over half a trillion dollars.[189] Bad decision making is expensive.

Consider the complexity of health care conditions and treatment options in addition to the increased competition for resources. It's easy to see how being health literate might come in handy in preventive care, managing a chronic illness or reacting to an acute or emergency medical event. Even if you live where health care is easily accessed, you can only have the best health outcomes by being health literate. There is a cost to be paid for its absence, which is why Americans' lack of health literacy is the third element of this perfect storm and the final ingredient in a potentially deadly recipe.

It was one thing to lack health literacy in the medical world of yesterday, with few options and adequate time for counsel if a decision had to be made. That is no longer the case. Care management challenges today may mean being confronted with a complex and/or long-term treatment plan, having insufficient time to seek expert input, being told needed resources are not available and/or not having any idea how to proceed. It's more critical than ever to achieve health literacy in preparation for what faces the system at large and you as an individual. Meandering along your health care journey without an information-gathering and decision-making skill set is no longer a viable plan for achieving the best health outcomes. Certainly, the picture of the future I've painted is not rosy, but buck up because you are about to see how those in charge have been preparing for the inevitable.

CHAPTER SIX

No worries. They've got this.

Policy makers and stakeholders have an eye-in-the-sky view of health care's past, present and future, and they're the default masterminds of the network poised to overcome challenges. Rising demographic demands, dwindling resources and a lack of health literacy. Exactly what is their plan to ensure patients and providers have the best possible health outcomes despite the perfect storm?

To be fair, not every problem has a solution. In viewing the perfect storm of health care, it's obvious some circumstances are unavoidable. Aging demographics, for instance. Ten years from now, every 50-year-old still living will be 60 years old, just as today's 70-year-olds will be 80. There's really no getting around that, at least not in a civilized society. First, there isn't an ice flow big enough to hold all the Boomers and second, we will not be going gently into that good night. As for the other challenges of this perfect storm, everything possible is being done to overcome them, right?

Here's an idea: Everybody get healthy!

Aging demographics is one thing, but America is also dealing with an epidemic of chronic illness and its demands for intense health care utilization. There are practical steps that could have been taken to stem the latter trend—and still could be—on both systems and individual levels. We know health literate lifestyles, preventive care and effective management of existing chronic conditions improve health outcomes. That is not debatable. The first Surgeon General to issue a *Report on Health Promotion and Disease Prevention* embraced that very notion with five goals, from healthy infants to healthy older adults. In the words of Joseph A. Califano, Jr., then Secretary of the U.S. Department of Health, Education and Welfare (nka HHS):

We are killing ourselves by our own careless habits. We are killing ourselves by carelessly polluting the environment. We are killing ourselves by permitting harmful social conditions to exist—conditions like poverty, hunger and ignorance—which destroy health, especially for infants and children.

It's a statement that would be apt in 2021, but was made in 1979. Within one year of the Secretary's recommendations, more than 300 national organizations and government entities convened and repackaged his directive as *Healthy People 1990,* the first initiative in a series that continues today. They turned the original five goals and ten subgoals into 226 health objectives for the following decade.[190] And the beat goes on. HHS generates a new *Healthy People* manifesto every ten years. By the time *Healthy People 2020* came along, there were 1,300 objectives.[191]

Are we reaching these goals for getting people healthy in America? Well, achievement rates range from 16 percent success for *Healthy People 1990* to 26 percent for *Healthy People 2020*, so you be the judge.[192] As an example, here are the results of just three objectives from *Healthy People 2020* focused on the health care issues of aging adults in America. That initiative came to a close on December 31, 2019:

- Increase the proportion of Medicare enrollees who use the *Welcome to Medicare benefit*: **The baseline rate was 6.4 percent / 2020 target objective of 7.0 percent / Achieved 6.8 percent.**

- Increase the proportion of registered nurses with a geriatric certification: **The baseline rate was 1.4 percent / 2020 target objective of 1.5 percent / Achieved .5 percent.**

- Reduce the rate of emergency department visits due to falls in older adults: **The baseline rate was 5,235.1 per 100,000 / 2020 target objective of 4,711.6 per 100,000 / Achieved 6,306.2 per 100,000.**[193]

There are only two conclusions to be drawn: We're setting the bar for healthy people in America inexplicably low and we still aren't reaching it. Yes, over the decades medical care has made monumental strides in extending life expectancy, along with incredible advances in disease management. Astonishing, really, and I have boundless respect for our health care professionals and their miraculous and tireless accomplishments, from researchers to direct care healers and caregivers. On the other hand, when it comes to policy makers' and stakeholders' efforts to foster wellness and health literacy, they get a big fat F minus.

For example, while the prevalence of smoking in all adults went from 1965's 42 percent to 15 percent in 2016, the *number* of smokers has been reduced by only 27 percent. We still have 38 million smokers in America and every day 1,600 teens try their first cigarette. While I am a big fan of free will and the right to make really stupid human decisions, smoking remains *the leading cause of preventable disease and death*—still the front-runner 57 years after the government launched its nationwide anti-smoking campaign.[194] That makes smoking a societal problem that warrants attention. Along the same lines, it may not surprise you to learn our level of daily physical activity has not increased since 2008, while the time spent on sedentary behavior (read: being sloths) has risen significantly.[195] The damage Americans did to their overall health during the pandemic hasn't even been factored in. No need to belabor this. You've had your first glimpse at the efforts and success of our institutional change agents in making Americans' lives healthier and fostering health literate decision making. Moving on, it's going to be tempting to avert your eyes, but don't.

If it weren't for the bad data, we'd have none at all

We know we can't change demographics. We know the health care system will be strained by the volume of medical care needed by an aging and chronically ill population—those are givens. We also know having so many providers age out of the system will be every bit as disruptive as all the high-maintenance patients aging in. Granted, we can't stop these evolving circumstances, but we still have an opportunity to prepare for their impact on health care delivery and access. (As an aside, this book focuses on health care, but the reality is that large segments of America's entire workforce will be retiring over the next few years, taking their expertise and mentoring with them. It's a demographic trend causing crippling shortages in every industry that's been in existence for more than 40 years, e.g., education, law enforcement, the skilled trades, the service industry, finance, insurance and the clergy. To name a few.)

Before any effective plan can be made, the impending danger has to be accurately and reliably quantified. In the past, America's policy makers have not been as proactive as we might wish—or, as we say here in Iowa, haven't managed to smell it before they stepped in it. Recall that halfway through the 18-year baby boom, the education experts were still stumped by where all those kids were coming from.[196] A similar failure to anticipate now leaves us with the unintelligible workforce projections you saw in Chapter Four. They are hardly the reliable guidance needed for effective planning, as providers or health care consumers. Surely policy makers and stakeholders know better because history has shown that projections have consequences.

As Boomers aged throughout the 1950s, 1960s and early 1970s, there was a growing consensus the United States needed to beef up its supply of physicians. They aimed to meet the needs of an expanding population, aid rural areas being abandoned for urban America and accommodate the creation and growth of Medicare and Medicaid, which both began in 1965.[197] Consequently, the government assisted communities in gaining a public health presence and incentivized medical school construction. It also escalated the funding of hospital residencies by the Centers for Medicare and Medicaid Services (CMS) for both foreign- and American-educated medical school graduates.[198] It worked.

It worked so well, in fact, that in 1981 the HHS-appointed Graduate Medical Education National Advisory Committee (GMENAC) projected we were heading for unacceptable physician *surpluses* of 70,000 by 1990 and 145,000 by 2000. They recommended reversing previous expansion efforts.[199] By 1992, another HHS advisory group, the Physician Payment Review Commission (PPRC), determined efforts weren't slowing things down fast enough.[200] In 1996, a study committee at the Institute of Medicine echoed that opinion,[201] and the HHS-appointed Council on Graduate Medical Education (COGME) also endorsed the sentiment. Congress then placed a cap on CMS-funded residencies in 1997, where it remained until December 2020.[202] Just to be clear, current policies on fostering an adequate health care workforce are at least partly founded on labor projections from *40 years ago*. Which is weird, because between the Worldwide Interweb and high-speed processors, we can assemble, analyze and disseminate a mind-boggling assortment of data in a nano second. Then why is it such a seemingly insurmountable task for agencies with full access to needed data to produce reliable evidence of how many health care workers we have, forecast how many we will need and then implement effective strategies?

Every health care professional who accepts Medicare or Medicaid has a National Provider Identifier (NPI). They don't get paid without it, so it seems simple enough to track the type and frequency of health care being provided to whom and by whom for a large segment of our population, some of the most frequent health care users. Here's that funny story I promised you. The Medicare Payment Advisory Commission (MedPAC) is a federal advisory group of 17 experts from within the health care finance and delivery industries; they've been providing Medicare analyses and policy advice to Congress since 1997. In October of 2019, the commissioners had to admit they had been including 46,000 doctors who don't really exist in the census of available PCPs. Instead of being PCPs, they're hospitalists so they only attend Medicare recipients who are, well, you know, hospitalized. Snap! Older and disabled patients were instantaneously ghosted by more than one fifth of the available primary care clinicians in America. Although MedPAC commissioners are confident this does not affect current health care access (because you can't miss what you only *thought* you had?), it "*underscores the Commission's concern about the future supply of PCPs*."[203] Doesn't this oversight make the *Health Professional Shortage Areas* (HPSAs) much more severe than previously acknowledged, since HRSA relies on data from CMS for those analyses?[204] Hmm . . .

That brings us back to the most recent HRSA projections forecasting about 300,000 out-of-work nurses by 2030, or maybe as early as 2025.[205] This research stands in stark contrast to the work of others who project *shortages* of 300,000 to 500,000 nurses occurring at the same time. One might be more inclined to give credence to HRSA's version of reality if federal agencies were known for producing up-to-date health care workforce data. They are not. For many years, health care stakeholders and bureaucrats themselves have pointed to the troubling lack of information on the number, type, location and work habits of health care professionals. Among others, critics include the Institute of Medicine, the U.S. Government Accountability Office, the Department of Veterans Affairs' Office of Inspector General, the Alliance for Health Reform, the

Robert Wood Johnson Foundation, AARP, the Association of Academic Health Centers, the American Academy of Nursing, the Council for the Advancement of Nursing Science and MedPAC.[206]

As a matter of fact, count HRSA—the agency responsible for collecting the data and making the projections—among those voicing frustration. Specifically, the stated mission of HRSA is to "*Identify and prioritize areas of current and future health care workforce needs and workforce training requirements through data-informed analysis and modeling.*" In HRSA's most recent projections for health care labor's largest segment, direct care workers, the staff regrets it can project only *demand*—but not *supply*—due to a lack of data.[207] Similarly, HRSA is making *no* supply/demand projections for medical and clinical lab technologists, EMTs, paramedics and community health workers because it lacks the data to do so.[208] And the most recent strategic plans for HHS and its subagency HRSA? They rely on seven- to twelve-year-old workforce data.[209] Honestly, how strategic can these plans really be?

Any stakeholders, policy makers or consumers hoping to use these forecasts for a little strategic planning of their own are out of luck. These so-called workforce projections from HRSA are no more insightful than those of the BLS, which disavow any opinion on whether future needs will be met. Talk about meaningless: In 2016, when HRSA looked ahead at patient access to psychiatrists, mental health counselors and family therapists for 2025, its best guess was shortages would be between 26,670 and 250,510 professionals. That's a helluva gap, and apparently that's as good as it gets "*In the absence of more specific data.*"[210] If only they had more data.

The Commission that never was

"*Woefully inadequate*" is how the Institute of Medicine (IOM) described our health care system's readiness to meet the needs of an aging population. That was in 2008. The National Academies is an independent, nonprofit organization chartered by Congress in 1863 to advise the federal government on scientific and technical matters. The IOM, nka the National Academy of Medicine (NAM), is just one part and was established by Congress in 1970 as the go-to source for research on biomedical science, medicine and health. Simply put, lawmakers and bureaucrats created the IOM to give them expert medical and health care advice. The 2008 study and report from IOM, "*Retooling for An Aging America*," went on to say, "*Immediate and substantial action is necessary by both public and private organizations to close the gap between the status quo and the impending needs of future older Americans.*" Okay, so it's not just you and me.

Really, the IOM could not have been more unambiguous in its assessment of America's aging demographics and its recommendations to meet the challenges of health care access in the coming decades. The first was to have the Bureau of Health

Professions, an HHS subagency, start making annual reports to Congress about its progress in addressing the coming health care workforce crisis.[211] There's no evidence that ever happened and the Bureau faded into oblivion in 2014. So that's a big *whatever.*[212]

Back to the strongly-worded findings and warnings from the IOM that "*The urgency for action cannot be overstated.*" I'm imagining IOM staff might have been somewhat disappointed when there was literally no bureaucratic response to their counsel. Maybe they even thought, "*If only there were an agency dedicated to compiling comprehensive and accurate health care workforce projections.*" But wait! Not long after the release of "*Retooling for An Aging America,*" the 2010 *Affordable Care Act* (ACA) established the National Health Care Workforce Commission (NHCWC) within HHS. As clearly stated in the ACA, the task of this commission is to collect and disseminate health care labor data needed to have "*a high-quality, readily accessible health care delivery system that meets the needs of patients and populations.*"[213] I know the IOM held great hope the NHCWC would carry out the "*bold and appropriate actions*" the IOM had identified as crucial to health care delivery. I know that because the IOM said so in 2011.[214] Certainly a commission such as the NHCWC would be a unique and invaluable resource for health care administrators, providers, big pharma, educators, manufacturers, policy makers, researchers, students, lawmakers and payers—not to mention health care consumers. I mean, who in the world would not think this information is critical to planning for and then achieving future health care access?

Apparently, members of the United States Congress. For over a decade they have failed to appropriate the relatively meager funds for the NHCWC to hold its first meeting and carry out its statutory duties under the ACA, which include providing an annual report to Congress. For well over a decade the NHCWC has had 15 fully-appointed members from throughout the health care industry, but its $3 million annual budget has never been approved or funded.[215] FYI, that's less than one millionth of total health care costs. It's also the same amount Congress appropriated for a turtle tunnel at Lake Jackson, Florida the year the *Affordable Care Act* was passed.[216]

To refresh your memory, when this workforce commission was created, HHS already had an entity with a similar mission focused exclusively on the physician workforce.[217] Formed in 1986, the Council on Graduate Medical Education (COGME) has been meeting regularly since then. You may recall it was their fear of a physician surplus that prompted the 1997 capping of medical student residencies. Well, in 2005, Council members began warning of an equally perilous physician *shortage* ahead and they now believe the current medical education model of residencies is insufficient to meet the changing needs of the nation. (Yes, the same funding model they moved to limit back in 1997.) COGME supports the formation of a new HHS committee to look into this situation and develop a strategic plan for graduate medical education.[218] Now I am confused, because that sounds a lot like what COGME is supposed to be doing.

Anyway, where might interested groups such as the NHCWC or COGME go to get the data and workforce projections needed to perform their assigned tasks, assuming they wanted to? Glad you asked. Along with the unfunded National Health Care Workforce Commission, the ACA also established the National Center for Health Workforce Analysis (NCHWA), to conduct "*analyses and projections on a wide range of health care occupations.*"[219] Unlike its counterpart commission, this subagency of HHS has been fully funded and staffed since 2010 and underwrites health care workforce research centers located at six universities.[220] Although its ACA mandate is to generate data for the work of the NHCWC, one can certainly understand no sense of urgency at the NCHWA, since the NHCWC has never held a meeting. Indeed, the last comprehensive study on the physician workforce under HHS's direction was conducted in 2006, using data from 2001.[221] More than 20 years ago. As for the nursing workforce, HHS/HRSA's January 2020 National Sample Survey of Registered Nurses was the first conducted in more than 13 years, though the website says it's done every four years (in fairness, it does say *approximately* every four years). However, it only addressed nurse workforce characteristics as of 2018 and provided no labor projections.[222]

Because you and I are people who now know stuff, we can judge for ourselves whether having 300,000 nurses, 250,000 social workers and 4,000 juvenile psychiatrists standing around with nothing to do seems like something that's likely to happen in 2030. Forget the fancy workforce simulation models, how about some common sense? Down the street from HHS, the BLS is projecting an additional 221,900 nursing jobs by 2029. One third of today's doctors and nurses will retire just when aging and chronically ill cohorts expand by far more than a third. Even with health care professionals entering the field, if only one of those events were certain to occur, it would be cause for concern. All three happening at the same time? Ruh-roh. In the future, if we look back and find reliance on HHS's forecast fails are the reason we suffer from life-threatening worker shortages, shame on the policy makers and leaders—elected and otherwise—now participating in this charade. Forecasts have consequences.

All this background by way of explaining why the HHS workforce projections for frontline health care professionals are so absurdly useless. It was also meant to clarify why the NCHWA doesn't give us reports on the supply/demand future for some of our most crucial health care professionals, such as direct care workers, medical and clinical lab technologists, EMTs, paramedics and community health workers. According to those charged with collecting that data: *Got no data.* We may have just uncovered a fourth element of this perfect storm: policy makers' and health care leaders' refusal to carry out their own mandates and prepare for what's obviously on its way.

Here come the magicians and the deniers

I would be remiss if I didn't include the viewpoint of those outside HHS who have also concluded no health care labor shortages lie ahead, and if they do, they can easily be overcome. Proposed solutions to adequately provide for greater numbers of aging and chronically ill patients include having nurse practitioners (NPs) and physician assistants (PAs) assume more of the duties now performed by primary care providers. It seems the Bureau of Labor Statistics agrees, as their staff recently cut the ten-year job growth projections for physicians by half and doubled numbers for NPs.[223] True, it stands to reason we will need fewer doctors if a bunch of us agree to not be seen by doctors, but marginalizing physicians' expertise isn't an optimal solution. I am not alone in believing that.[224] It's reminiscent of the 1950s. Upon realizing the education system needed 800,000 more elementary school teachers than were available, policy makers simply lowered teacher certification requirements. Then along came Sputnik . . .

Then there's the proposal to just make the health care environment more pleasant so doctors will work longer. It was prompted by survey results in which more than one third of physicians said they would put off retirement if their work load were cut in half. Reasoning then follows we can keep doctors working longer and solve the potential provider shortage with NPs and PAs assuming care for half of the doctors' existing patients.[225] Wait just a darn minute. I thought NPs and PAs were already the remedy for the additional aging and chronically ill patients? So this plan calls for them to actually be in two places at once, tending to the increased patient load *and* covering for doctors who want more time off? Although quantum particles can be in two places at once, NPs and PAs cannot. Also, nurses choosing to become NPs over the past decade have already reduced the nursing workforce by 80,000.[226] If you've ever played Musical Chairs, this will be a lot like that, except when the music stops, someone goes without health care.

It's been suggested we address the HPSA geographic shortages by requiring newly-minted doctors to work in underserved areas for two years. First, I'm fairly certain forced labor is illegal in this country. I also think we would discover that while young doctors are presently free to work anywhere, they don't want to go to those places. Another idea being floated is the hope for a well-timed recession. The resulting drop in personal wealth would then encourage nurses to delay retirement, as seems to have been the case in 2008. No. How about the proposition that there really is no shortage—doctors are just bad at time management? It's a 2017 theory using 1986 census figures, so I'm not sure what to make of it,[227] but based on all I've read, seen and heard, uh, no.

I'll end by returning to the idea that never gets old: Let's just have patients take better care of themselves. Although it is certainly a worthy goal to have everyone be healthier, 40 years of *Healthy People* initiatives have proven that those positioned to promote such a concept have never managed to succeed, not even close. Second, as we've already seen, if people were to become healthier, impliedly they would live longer, which ultimately puts an even greater strain on existing resources. A nonstarter.

Of course, I was kidding when I said "*They've got this*"

As we witness policy makers' denial and/or lack of preparation for what's over the horizon, there is little doubt that developing and implementing strategies for our self-preservation will be shouldered by us, not them. Afterall, these are the same folks who consistently refuse to authorize a lousy $9 million a year for needed geriatric and end-of-life specialists;[228] have failed to properly oversee agencies charged with preserving resources; and—my personal favorite—have never appropriated the funds needed to assemble vital health care workforce data, a statutory mandate of their creation. Pleas to increase funding for residencies have been ignored for so long the proposed *Resident Physician Shortage Reduction Act of 2007* was last known as the *Resident Physician Shortage Reduction Act of 2021*. Then voila! The *Consolidated Appropriations Act of 2021*, which became law on December 27, 2020, included additional Medicare-funded residencies over a 5-year period. Albeit only 1,000 of them, it's the first meaningful increase in this Medicare funding since 1997, which is something.[229] When you think about it, those with unfettered access to a primary care physician and specialists where they work would naturally struggle with the concept of shortages. Yes, the Attending Physician of the U.S. Congress provides routine and emergency care to all congressmen, senators and Supreme Court justices for an annual per head fee of $627.[230]

Something to keep in mind as you read further is the meaning of the term *stakeholder*. The dictionary says it's a person with a vital interest in what's going on. In any discussion of health care access, you'd think *stakeholder* would include those whose very lives depend on available and positive health outcomes. Nevertheless, anytime a mission statement mentions *stakeholders*, it most definitely doesn't include you and me. Who can we turn to for advocacy?

I've previously mentioned a few of the health care-related citizen councils (COGME, MedPAC, etc.) among the bounty of public/private task forces, summits, round tables, commissions, consortiums, compendiums and advisory boards formed over the life of our nation. The stated intent of these federal advisory committees is to afford the public "*an opportunity to provide input into a process that may form the basis for government decisions*." Through a tradition in place since the Washington administration, we've invited nonbureaucrats to offer direct input to those who make the laws and regulations. Advisory committees are occupied by representatives from business, academia and local governments. They are meant to contribute expertise, opinions and recommendations to policy makers and bureaucrats. For decades, many outsiders have voiced concerns over the failure of these groups to reflect the public good, their inefficient duplication of official functions and a general lack of transparency.[231] Well, there are now nearly 1,000 federal advisory committees with more than 74,000 appointees (that number has grown by 3,225 since FY 2019), at an annual taxpayer cost of $360 million.[232]

It just so happens that over one fourth of these federal advisory committees lie within one agency, the U.S. Department of Health and Human Services (HHS).[233] This would seem to present rare opportunities to mine industry expertise in addressing challenges to health care access. Afterall, HHS's $1.4 trillion annual budget controls these agencies:

- Administration for Children and Families (ACF)
- Administration for Community Living (fka Administration on Aging, the Office on Disability, and the Administration on Developmental Disabilities)
- Agency for Healthcare Research and Quality (AHRQ)
- Agency for Toxic Substances and Disease Registry (ATSDR)
- Centers for Disease Control and Prevention (CDC)
- Centers for Medicare & Medicaid Services (CMS)
- Food and Drug Administration (FDA)
- Health Resources and Services Administration (HRSA)
- Indian Health Service (IHS)
- National Institutes of Health (NIH)
- Substance Abuse and Mental Health Services Administration (SAMHSA)[234]

Who better than the members of those 260 HHS advisory committees to speak for the end users of all things health care and to ask the tough questions about anticipating and preparing for the future of health care? And, naturally, to contribute invaluable wisdom on the formulation and implementation of solutions?

Here's the thing. Appointees for all federal advisory committees are chosen from within the professions and organizations directly impacted by the respective agency's regulations; academia who subsist on government contracts and funding of research; and entities lobbying for and consulting with associated special interests. In limited instances, statutory charters call for members of the public, or groups claiming to represent them, to be included. However, even when mandated by law those assigned seats at the table may or may not be filled. And it bears mentioning that 80 percent of the 6,776 advisory committee meetings held in FY 2020 were not open to the public. Ninety-four percent of the closed meetings had to do with grant application reviews—the laying on of taxpayers' funds.[235] The late Justice Arthur Goldberg said it best: "*If Columbus had an advisory committee, he would probably still be at the dock.*"

You've seen how deficient health care leaders have been in gathering data and making the policies needed to prepare for health care's perfect storm. The nature of their plan to ensure the best health outcomes for us in the coming years and decades is painfully obvious, i.e., they don't have one. Now let's see how this perfect storm will impact the individual, someone just like you—and me.

PART TWO

Where does this leave us?

CHAPTER SEVEN

What happens when you take it personally

Anytime stakeholders and policy makers talk big, incomprehensible numbers—like total health care expenditures—it's a 10,000 foot view of health care. But for patients and advocates at ground level, the perspective is very different. This approaching storm is like any other: The sooner we know what's coming, the better we can prepare.

I live in tornado country and some might not admit it, but when we hear a warning siren, we run to the largest plate glass window or out onto the deck. As you can imagine, what we observe at ground level is a lot different than what's being viewed on the Super-Uber-Doppler screen. That's *perspective,* like hearing about $3.8 trillion in health care spending or knowing 150 million of the most demanding patients imaginable are crowding the system or recognizing two million doctors and nurses are planning their mass exodus. After hearing just a few *millions*, *billions* and *trillions*, there's a serious risk of desensitization. We soon forget that every supersized statistic is reflective of countless individuals, folks like you and me trying to navigate our medical journeys, and health care practitioners pushing through the work day. The merit of largescale statistics shrinks when you're in an acute medical crisis, managing a chronic illness or seeking comfort at the end of life. Let's just say that if your doctor voices concern about your EKG, you will be less focused on *What's the job market look like for cardiologists, doc?* and more on *How soon can you get me in to see one?* Suddenly, macro demographic trends get very personal.

Not everyone is going to have the same health care experience—the pandemic made that clear—and why would they? Chronically ill versus generally healthy, young versus old, high income versus impoverished, insured versus uninsured, literate versus illiterate, rural versus urban. That last category serves as a useful illustration. In Chapter Four, I mentioned the closure of 130 rural hospitals over the past ten years and the implication for those communities. *Reduced access* sounds like a minor inconvenience but it's really a matter of life or death. Americans who live in rural settings are more likely than those in urban areas to die from the five leading causes of death, and that's nationwide, not just in communities without a hospital. For those living in rural areas, even unintentional injury deaths number 50 percent more than in large cities. That comes from a higher risk for car accidents, opioid overdoses and the distance from trauma centers and specialized care.[236] In spite of the wide gaps between available workforce projections, if you read the fine print, you'll see every one agrees health care access in the United States is *geographically challenged.* Inequities are obvious across the country and even within states. We can see that America's health care crisis is not just about being able to pay for health care, it is also about having resources located for timely access. (So, besides the income tax rate and average temperature, the location and quality of health care should be considerations when choosing your retirement community.) HRSA says Iowa barely meets half its need for primary care physicians, and I'm not questioning that, but everything's fine where I'm at. My PCP is 15 minutes away and there are specialists even closer. On the other hand, I know Iowans who must drive hours for needed care. As we consider what a typical health care journey might look like in the midst of a perfect storm, keep in mind the autonomous perspectives we bring to these experiences. Individual coping skills and system-wide plans both need to reflect that diversity.

Whether prompted by injury or illness, the adventure usually starts in a clinic or emergency department. First, we'll hope you survive long enough to arrive. Unless their financial situation dramatically improves, between 20 and 40 percent of the remaining 2,000 rural hospitals are at an immediate or high risk of shutting down. They can't afford to keep up with medical technology because they lack the capital; they lack the capital because they can't adequately compete for patients and providers, partly because their technology is outdated.[237] It's a dangerous cycle with a direct bearing on health care access for residents of smaller communities, all 46 million of them.

Because you're now familiar with the demographics of aging and chronic illness, you realize how they impact the use of health care-related resources, reducing availability for everyone. Each year, almost half of those aged 60 and older seek emergency care—it's 86 percent for those aged 90 and over.[238] Although younger people may not be getting annual checkups, they have a much higher risk of having an accident than other cohorts until age 45. When they arrive at the emergency department, they'll be competing with their parents and grandparents for medical attention.

I think we can all agree time is finite. If a doctor sees 24 patients a day and gives each one 20 minutes, he can serve a panel of about 2,000. As aging and chronically ill patients visit more often, something has to give. In fact, if a panel mimics the general population, as the proportion of seniors grows, a larger number of the younger patients will have to go elsewhere. That's basic math—appointments will already be snarfed by the frequent fliers. Unless, of course, the doctor decides to put a quota on chronically ill, older and less profitable patients (read: Medicare and Medicaid recipients), which many are already doing.[239] Hey, in what business does it not make sense to focus on clients who pay the highest rates with the least amount of paperwork, especially when the waiting room is never empty?

To begin with, limited resources cause longer waits to see a provider, which can delay diagnoses, diminish positive health outcomes and leave doctors without the time to discuss healthy living options or preventive care.[240] Failing to either properly manage chronic conditions or coordinate the treatment of comorbidities is a hazard on both individual and systemic levels. Unnecessary and potentially dangerous duplications jeopardize patient safety and deter the efficient delivery of health care. COVID-19 was a vivid illustration of how a system-wide allocation of resources impacts individuals. It is impossible to accurately measure the harm and loss of life that resulted from delays in treating noncoronavirus medical conditions while all available labor and assets were directed at the pandemic.[241] People failed to seek needed medical care for acute and emergency events because they were terrified to enter a clinic or hospital, assuming that was an option. Delays were commonplace for nonemergency medicine, such as preventive care, diagnostic tests, cancer treatments and heart procedures, as clinics and outpatient surgery centers were shuttered. No one was prepared to provide for secondary medical services and prevent life-altering consequences during a pandemic.

And careful what we wish for. Only about one in four Medicare beneficiaries makes an Annual Wellness Visit to a primary care provider.[242] If we encourage consumers to focus more on preventive care and—OMG—we succeed, how would the system handle another 48 million appointments every year? As it is, less than two thirds of those without a chronic condition have a primary care physician.[243] It's tough to wrap your head around how many more doctors would be needed if everyone appreciated the advantages of being in a patient panel. It also makes the point that you will definitely have trouble accessing a PCP if you don't already have one.

Let's say that trip to the clinic or emergency department gets you admitted to the hospital. (The transition from the emergency department to a room has its own set of issues, so Chapter 16 is devoted to the hazards of the *care handoff* in various settings.) Sixty percent of all nurses work in hospitals. Those 221,900 nursing jobs being added by 2029? BLS projects the fastest growth will be in long term care facilities, rehabilitation hospitals and outpatient chronic disease treatment centers.[244] As time goes on, we'll see how that impacts the nursing shortages already being felt in hospitals. An unanswered call button is frustrating, the lack of staff needed to keep a hospital room hygienic is hazardous, but as concerning is the human link missing from the chain of risk management, e.g., when there is no longer a second set of eyes to double-check medications. Insufficient staff to properly oversee medical care correlates with higher readmissions, greater risks for hospital-acquired urinary tract and surgical site infections and patient falls.[245] Considering existing shortages in the direct care worker industry (personal care aides, home health aides, nursing assistants and orderlies), you may find that your expectations for room and patient hygiene will not be met as they used to be.

If you're sick enough to be hospitalized, better hope you have a friend or family member to oversee your care and step in when no staff is available.

You're now in a hospital room and a person enters claiming to be your doctor, but you don't recognize her even a little. Your medical condition is not to blame. You've never met before. While hospitalized, your attending physician is likely to be a *hospitalist* and not your beloved PCP. A hospitalist works full-time treating patients who don't have personal physicians or whose doctors don't make hospital rounds. They're trained in general medicine or have a board certified specialty, such as internal medicine or pediatrics. Among hospitalists, we have even more subspecialties, such as *nocturnists* (work at night), *weekendists* (work on weekends) and *triagists* (evaluate patients for potential treatment and/or admission). This dramatic change in the delivery of inpatient care may make more efficient use of clinicians' time and also has the potential of improving the consistency, availability and quality of hospital medicine. However, it does create a unique challenge for provider-patient communication. (The good news is, we now know there are 46,000 more hospitalists available than we previously thought!) If hospitalized, there's a chance you may lack full decision-making capacity, either because of your condition or medication. Without an advocate by your side, how can a hospitalist just meeting you spot inaccuracies in your electronic medical record or realize what's missing? Or be familiar with your personal and treatment goals? Or recognize any existing hearing, visual, cognitive or mobility issues? All good questions. There's much more in Chapter Twelve about how to overcome these obstacles to getting the best care while hospitalized.

Being fully informed in order to make health literate decisions throughout your hospital stay is key to having the best health outcomes. That's always been true, but increased competition for resources makes it even more important. We should assume the specialists we rely on while hospitalized, such as radiologists, therapists and lab technicians, will not escape workforce shortages, which may cause delays in accessing tests and treatments. If you haven't been in or around a hospital recently, this is not yesterday's health care journey. Chapters Eleven through Sixteen focus on how to make the most of available resources in any health care setting, while preserving your rights to informed consent, autonomy and safety.

Once ready to leave the hospital, you will likely spend time discussing post-discharge care options and recommendations for medical and caregiving needs. This *handoff* from one level of care to another or from one provider to another is viewed as one of the most dangerous times in a health care journey. Whether you meet with a social worker, attending physician or discharge nurse, you'll have limited time to absorb vital information about the next care steps to be taken. Communication failures surrounding the treatment plan, caregiving needs, medications, specialist referrals and therapies are a primary contributing cause of unintended and harmful consequences, known as *adverse events*.[246] Treasure any time with a social worker because it's another occupation losing ground. The social work industry is projected to suffer a shortfall of 195,000 employees by 2030 due to retirements and burnout.[247] Or a surplus of 250,000?

If you do require some level of caregiving at discharge, how will that need be met? Most persons hope to stay for as long as possible in the home they know and love. There certainly was a time when the frail or disabled lived with and were cared for by family members until an unavoidable move to a nursing home, if ever. Today, anyone needing hands-on support is less likely to have an available live-in caregiver—there's no one else in the house to be of assistance. That's partly because single-person households have gone from one in eight to nearly one in every three over the past 60 years.[248] Also, staying in the home is only feasible if the physical environment is functional and home health care assistance is available. Throughout this decade, the number of potential caregivers will increase by only one percent, while those aged 80 and older needing assistance will rise by 79 percent.[249] Don't misunderstand, more than 53 million persons are providing unpaid care to another, which is great.[250] At the same time, there are an estimated 13 million adults with no family member or friend available to even speak for them, let alone provide direct caregiving assistance.[251]

This brings us to a statistical concept analogous to the *dependency ratio*. When we compare those aged 45 to 64 to those aged 80 and older, we get the *caregiver support ratio*. It's a measurement of the number of persons in a population available to care for the elderly. As Boomers entered their prime caregiving years from 1990 to 2020, the caregiver support ratio rose, made up of both professionals and unpaid family members. However, as the oldest Boomers turn 80 in 2026, that trend will sharply reverse, shrinking from 2010's ratio of seven caregivers for every aged person, to four caregivers by 2030 and to three by 2050.[252] As for paid providers, direct care workers serve in many settings besides clients' homes. They're in hospitals, skilled nursing facilities, continuing care and assisted living communities, dementia care centers and rehabilitation clinics. Although about half are employed as home health workers, it's still projected we'll need over 650,000 additional employees in that category by 2029 to keep up with increased demand and job separations.[253]

Over the next 15 years, we will grow to have 17 million households of older adults where at least one person has limited mobility. Unfortunately, only four percent of America's single family homes offer one-story living, extra-wide doorways and zero-step thresholds.[254] On the other hand, there are now lifestyle options that didn't exist not so very long ago: independent living, assisted living, memory units, rehabilitation hospitals and a whole menu of professional home services. These caregiving and living accommodations sprouted from necessity and demand as families shrank and values shifted. Will we have sufficient age-sensitive and mobility-appropriate resources? It's wise to have realistic expectations about available choices.

You may be headed for a nursing facility for more intense assistance or full-time rehabilitation. Once you reach age 65, there's a 70 percent chance you'll use long-term services and supports (LTSS) during your lifetime. LTSS include assistance with daily personal care, such as nutrition, medication management, transportation, mobility, dressing and bathing. Odds are one in three a senior will reside in a nursing home for at least 90 days at some point, and the risk is four times as high for those with dementia.[255]

And what will you find when you get there? Federal regulations require sufficient staff to oversee care, provide resident safety and assure overall patient well-being.[256] In real life that translates to nurse-to-patient ratios ranging from one-to-18 on best-staffed days and one-to-30 patients on worst-staffed days. On weekends, those increase to 20 patients (best) and 39 patients (worst) for every nurse on duty. As for direct care workers—the people we depend on for one-on-one personal care, mobility support and safety—there are nine to 14 residents assigned to a single worker on weekdays and ten to 17 during weekends. The ability to maintain even this questionably adequate level of staffing is directly tied to whether those 1.3 million *additional* direct care worker jobs are filled by the end of this decade.[257] As always, vigilant oversight by the patient's advocate—if there is one—is crucial to receiving acceptable attention at any level of health care.

If you want to hire care assistance, this gives you an idea of what these services cost. Medicare, Medicaid, private health insurance or long-term care insurance coverage may apply to some or all of these costs, depending on circumstances:

- $150 to $184 per day for home health care (8-hour day, more for skilled nursing)
- $75 per day for adult day care
- $4,050 to $4,300 per month for assisted living, plus costs for extra services
- $5,300 per month for memory care for persons with cognitive issues
- $7,400 to $8,821 per month for residential nursing care[258]

It's a brave new world out there in health care land. This is not the supply/demand crisis of Christmas 1961 that left millions of little girls suffering the agony of no Barbie under the tree. No ma'am. These are real people, not statistical cohorts. What we've seen in this chapter is how the shortages inherent in health care's perfect storm already impact accessibility and logistics, a trend that will accelerate over time. Even having the means to pay for health care does not guarantee its availability, and being on a waiting list is not the same as receiving care. If you've ever considered how practitioners are reacting to what's happening in health care today and what promises to materialize in the future, you are about to find out.

CHAPTER EIGHT

How health care professionals are prepping

It isn't only patients who must adapt in order to survive, and don't think everyone on the provider side is asleep at the wheel. In fact, sensing what this perfect storm means to the quality of their work environment, many health care professionals are already adjusting how they practice medicine. The choices they make, both proactive and reactive, are about to rock our world.

Not to brag, but I have had great doctors. Incredibly talented, exceptional diagnosticians who practice the art of healing with compassion and empathy. One of their more appealing qualities has been my ability to see them when I need to, which is major because *having* a doctor and *having access* to a doctor are no longer synonymous. Twenty years ago, when I began learning and writing about the future of health care in America, 2030 was referred to as *The Wall.* Those of us peering ahead felt certain the end of this decade is when the clash of high demand with low supply would resemble a train hitting the side of a mountain. Little did we know.

Observing a group of people celebrating their 50th birthdays, we can say with 100 percent certainty that ten years later, those still living will turn 60. Supported by data gathering and statistical analyses of past and present cohorts, we can even make educated guesses about the group's use of health care resources and overall survival rate. In reality, projecting demographics is easy work compared to visualizing the future medical conditions or life decisions of a single individual. The same is true of health care professionals. When characterizing their roles in the medical melodrama to come, one of many underlying assumptions has been that they would cooperate by continuing to do what they've always done until reaching their mid-60s. As we are beginning to realize, that's not happening.

Even if you haven't yet experienced it first-hand, you now recognize the impending impact of health care labor shortages. Policy makers and stakeholders may be stoically denying any looming crisis in health care access, but I can assure you practitioners cannot and are not. The demands of how we deliver, pay for and keep records of medical care in America have turned the tide on health care professionals' job descriptions and job satisfaction. Throughout the coming chapters, we'll focus on how we can aim for best outcomes as health care consumers. First, let's consider what it's like for those who spend half their lives immersed in the delivery side of the system and reflect on how this perfect storm is affecting providers' peace of mind and ability to practice. You and I are naturally focused on picking the best available professionals to be our medical experts and caregivers, but stepping outside ourselves for a moment, have we ever pictured not being chosen as a patient? How are providers responding to today's work environment and what's to come?

In case you're considering the glamorous life of a healer . . .

What's the investment required to become a doctor? Talk about an evolving business model. Forty years ago, medical school cost about $32,000. Twenty years later, it was closer to $200,000, leaving a new doctor with $150,000 in debt. Today, it's more like $290,000 to attend medical school, and then graduate with student loans of $200,000 and more.[259] Besides the outlay in money and time, consider the expectations for providers. They're required to stay current with a medical knowledge base estimated to double every 73 days,[260] and the International Classification of Diseases 10th Revision of 2015 had 19 times as many medical procedure codes and five times as many diagnosis codes as in 1979.[261] In truth, doctors spend only one fourth to one half of their day directly caring for patients, after electronic recordkeeping duties and an additional two to three hours of nonclinical paperwork each evening.[262] No, probably not what the medical school recruiter promised.

And where does revenue come from? One hundred years ago, an average family's annual medical expenses were only about $100, so the more pressing financial concern was going without earnings during an illness. An enterprising person created *sickness insurance*, which covered lost income to the family in case of the wage-earner's illness or injury. Health insurance as we now know it began with prepaid hospitalization plans in the early 1930s and then included physicians' services in the 1940s. It eventually became today's system of commercial and government insurers collecting premiums and paying institutional and individual providers on a fee-for-services basis. Health care practitioners and facilities negotiate fee schedules directly with commercial payers and choose whether to accept payment from government health insurance programs such as Medicare, Medicaid and the State Children's Health Insurance Program (CHIP). As of 2019, only 9.2 percent of all Americans were not covered by some form of health insurance.[263]

For hospitals, private insurance plans pay 150 to 400 percent of what Medicare pays for the same care. For physicians' services and procedures, it's 11 to 100 percent more than rates paid by Medicare.[264] In other words, Medicare patients bring in only one fourth to two thirds of the revenue generated by privately insured patients or those paying cash for the same medical treatment. The effect on the bottom line is simple math: Once a patient qualifies for Medicare by being permanently disabled or turning

65, the income generated by their clinic visits and hospitalizations is less, a lot less. And don't forget, there are at least ten thousand new Medicare insureds added to those rolls every day. Ergo, as the age of a doctor's patient panel goes up, the revenue stream goes down. Since Medicare was introduced in 1965, we've been a spread sheet away from reliably predicting how demographics directly affect the income side of the American health care business model. And yet . . .

Then there's the cost of doing business. Revenue doesn't just appear once services are rendered, not like when patients paid the doctor, then got reimbursed by the insurer. For providers, the cost of the billing and insurance-related part of health care—filing and then chasing claims—is estimated at $282 billion per year. About one third of all health care costs are annual administrative expenses, between $812 billion and $1.1 trillion.[265]

Mad as hell and not taking it anymore

Policy makers and stakeholders have been reinventing the modern system of health care delivery and payment for decades, creating a labyrinth now dependent on electronic health records (EHRs) and the input of more than 141,000 EHR codes. There's just one thing missing from these puppet masters' well-oiled plans: You can't make health care professionals do what they are no longer willing to do. All modern technology aside, providers are humans and sometimes people say *no more*.

Burnout is the reaction of an individual medical professional to the challenges of health care logistics. Plaguing doctors, nurses, dentists, physician assistants, direct care workers, nurse practitioners, pharmacists, administrative staff, emergency workers—really, anyone involved in health care—burnout is long-term job stress on steroids. The most common signs are emotional exhaustion, a low sense of job satisfaction, cynicism and detachment. Of course, that's how burnout is expressed on the intellectual and emotional levels. The more subtle but potentially deadlier risks are for cardiovascular disease, Type 2 diabetes, prolonged fatigue, headaches, respiratory problems, substance abuse, depression and suicide. And all that's in addition to the occupational hazards of musculoskeletal injuries, needle sticks, biohazards and disease transmission.[266]

The percentage of providers who admit to feelings of burnout is no blip on the radar. Studies show eight in ten physicians sometimes, often or always experience those feelings. One third to one half of nurses and physicians and 40 percent of physician assistants admit to having substantial symptoms.[267] And these studies were conducted before health care workers' trial by fire throughout the pandemic.

Careful who you seek out for encouragement if your child shows interest in being a doctor. Only one fourth to one half of surveyed physicians would recommend the practice of medicine to their own children.[268] These elders of the industry are the work horses of medicine; in the middle of the pack, age-wise, they possess the lion's share of practical experience and wisdom. Just as they reach their peak in terms of performance and compensation, stress diminishes their productivity, along with their ability and willingness to lead and mentor younger health care professionals.

When burnout pushes providers to reduce workloads or change career paths, there are quantifiable costs to the health care system from recruitment and lost revenue while jobs remain unfilled and new practitioners get up to speed. Estimates are two to three times a physician's annual salary, or $500,000 to $1,000,000 per vacancy. Industry-wide, yearly expenses for turnover and reduced output are about $5 billion, with some estimates as high as $31 billion, not including potential lost revenue of an additional $28 billion. Stanford Medicine studied their own staff and found that without interventions to prevent likely losses from burnout, projected costs over two years would range from $15.5 million to $55.5 million.[269] One institution. Financial and administrative burdens may materialize long before a provider leaves. While still practicing, those suffering from burnout make more mistakes and may even cause deaths through medical errors, leading to malpractice suits. Their patients may have higher infection rates, longer recovery times and reduced patient satisfaction. Damage to the institution's reputation and brand loyalty can result from clinicians performing below par. All that can lead to lowered reimbursements and reduced revenue.[270]

One way to deal with a stressful environment is to reduce one's exposure. In fact, many doctors are willing to make less money in exchange for more free time. Almost half say they are planning to change their work load in some manner in one to three years, e.g., cut back on hours, become a hospitalist, work part-time or change business models. There's still much to learn about the pandemic's impact on the health care workforce, but we already know 8 percent of physicians closed their practices as a result of COVID-19; 4 percent, or 8,000 doctors, plan to close their practice within 12 months of a July 2020 survey; and approximately 134,000 doctors will change their practice in a way that disrupts patient care, at least temporarily, in the near future.[271] With 80 percent claiming their practice is already at full capacity or overextended, one in five doctors intends to reduce clinic hours, and half to nearly three quarters are thinking about quitting all together. Almost 50 percent of nurses have considered leaving the profession.[272] This is so not good for us.

Some health care professionals seek greater financial benefits to offset burdens. Finding the compensation sweet spot happens when a student chooses a medical specialty or an established professional considers a mid-career switch. Average pay for cardiologists, orthopedic surgeons, gastroenterologists and urologists is $200,000 to $400,000 more than a family physician earns. For all specialties, average annual pay is $100,000 more than for all primary care physicians. Is it surprising that from 2002 to

2018, the number of medical students choosing general internal medicine dropped from 23 to 11 percent, adding to the primary care provider shortages we're already facing?[273]

Even in this day and age and even in a profession centered on human needs, acknowledging the mental health and emotional issues associated with burnout carries a stigma that discourages many practitioners from seeking help. Although some providers consider prescribed drugs for anxiety or depression, others self-medicate with unhealthy behaviors and substance abuse.[274] Talk about a perfect storm. It's no wonder an alarming percentage of health care professionals are questioning their career choices. Today's providers have practicable and lucrative options. I'll let you judge whether the alternatives that seem beneficial to providers are also good for patients.

Who is that in the white coat?

Robert Wachter, MD first used the term *hospitalist* in a 1996 article in the New England Journal of Medicine. It marked the launch of a medical specialty now grown to 57,000 providers employed by 75 percent of U.S. hospitals. Although nurse practitioners and physician assistants may also identify as hospitalists, the term usually refers to a doctor who is a patient's attending physician and manages care during hospitalization, from the emergency department to discharge. Almost 40 percent of doctors now work directly for a hospital or in a practice at least partially owned by a hospital or health system. In fact, the share of physicians in private practice has dropped below 50 percent for the first time since tracking began in 2012.[275]

Initially I had doubts about being cared for by someone other than my trusted primary care provider, but research—both empirical and anecdotal—suggests having a doctor on full-time hospital duty promises greater efficiency, improved patient satisfaction and better health outcomes, if properly executed.[276] Being a hospitalist is not without its own stresses, but in general it pays about $36,000 more than a primary care provider's annual compensation, and hospitalists also have opportunities for teaching and research in addition to providing direct patient care.[277] Hospitalist medicine is but one of several options for those seeking alternatives to the traditional medical business model.

Sure, I'd pay extra for cutsies!

Let's revisit the ideal patient panel size, where we can again credit the Boomers with bending medicine's economic curve. A panel is the total number of individual patients seen by a clinician over the past 12 to 18 months. It's been traditionally estimated at about 2,500 patients, even as high as 3,000.[278] That's just silly. An average of only three visits per year per person—demographically outdated—requires a ten- to 11-hour work day, plus off duty computer screen time. Furthermore, patients would be seen for only ten minutes each, when you allow for transition time between appointments, and that ten minutes would include all data input. One source even speculates a doctor would need 21.7 hours per day to provide recommended care to a panel of 2,500 patients.[279]

Doctors actually see 20 or fewer patients per day, which is still only 24 minutes per patient in an eight-hour day—and that 24-minute visit includes transition time and charting time. Oh, and no lunch break.[280] (I can tell you my doctor thinks he's getting off easy if I stay for just 24 minutes.) Considering clinicians' practice styles and specialties, it's tough to nail down a universally acceptable panel size, but we know this: Whatever combination of factors contribute, when a doctor becomes *over-empaneled*, provider burnout goes up and patient access goes down.

What about panel revenue? For more than five decades, health care's business model has depended on private health insurance to make up for Medicare and Medicaid's low reimbursement schedules. It's easy to see how demographics and the rising costs of getting paid work to shrink net income when the number of older patients grows. Here's the question: As a patient, would you be willing to pay more to be first in line for appointments or get right into the specialist you need to see? How about paying extra to see a doctor who has time for an engaged and expansive patient-provider relationship and is willing to be an overall care manager? Is it possible smaller panels would appeal to patients as well as providers, even if out-of-pocket costs are greater?

Welcome to *concierge medicine,* a health care business model already practiced by between 6,000 and 20,000 doctors. Patients pay an out-of-pocket monthly membership fee of $125 to $200 (which may be adjusted for the patient's age) to receive premium care and priority treatment, in addition to other insurance-covered services. There may also be per-visit fees. (There are *boutique practices* charging up to $80,000 a year for a family, but that model doesn't work for most folks.) For instance, a concierge patient may receive a comprehensive executive annual physical, shorter wait times, longer visits, quicker access to specialists, use of patient-provider communication technology and care coordination of hospitalizations and multiple specialists. And if you've been missing the Doc Welbys of this world, dare I say there's even the possibility of house calls and 24/7 access to the doctor's cell phone?

At 150 to 600 clients, depending on fee structure and the services provided, a concierge patient panel is a fraction of the theoretical 2,500 patients. Do the math: 600 patients paying $200 a month is $1,440,000 in annual membership fee revenue. And the switch to concierge medicine seems to lift attitudes along with compensation. One study shows more than 80 percent of these practitioners rate their morale as positive, citing strong patient relationships as the most satisfying result of being in a concierge practice. Seventy-five percent of concierge doctors would choose the medical profession if they had it to do again.[281] The business side of concierge medicine can be more complicated for providers who accept patients with Medicare coverage because they can't charge an additional fee for any treatment already included in Medicare's schedule of services.[282] Which is why concierge medicine is sometimes referred to as *premium care*: the services it offers go above and beyond standard care.

For providers who want to entirely avoid the preapproval and collection work associated with insurance reimbursement—and that's more than 40 percent of surveyed doctors—there is the *direct primary care* (DPC) model. As in concierge medicine, the DPC client pays a monthly or annual fee for a defined set of services, but DPC providers accept *no* payments from third party payers, such as commercial health insurers or Medicare/Medicaid. Although 70 to 80 percent of DPC practices have been in operation for less than three to four years (as of 2018), the American Academy of Family Physicians estimates nearly 8,000 members are either in a DPC clinic or are transitioning to it. Dominated by family medicine physicians, these practices have average panels of 345 patients, with an average target of 596.[283]

From a business standpoint, the obvious advantage of DPC is the elimination of regulatory and administrative obstacles to getting paid, including obtaining preapprovals and the data entry of complex treatment codes. Gone is the expense of employees dedicated to account receivables and filing/chasing insurance claims. For both patients and providers, the intrinsic benefits are similar to those of a concierge practice: increased access with more personalized and comprehensive care. Available DPC services may include laboratory tests and the dispensing of medications, and monthly DPC membership fees are typically less than concierge medicine, from $50 to $75 for individuals. Clients still need health care insurance coverage for specialists, hospitalization or diagnostic tests outside the scope of DPC services, but may be able to choose a less comprehensive and lower cost insurance plan. By the way, a clinician can also choose to have a *hybrid* practice consisting of both DPC and fee-for-service panels.

With more than half of doctor visits made to PCPs, innovative care models have appeal for employers seeking to self-insure employees' basic health care needs.[284] Millennials outnumber Boomers and are comparably healthier, upping their value as membership patients. At the same time, high-maintenance patients are attracted to this concept if willing and able to pay for time-sensitive care. With more than twice the number of seniors as in 1980 and 55 percent more than in 2000,[285] there's a larger pool of customers to draw from in establishing a patient panel of profitable size.

Traditional fee-for-services payment models that thrive on the number of patients seen in a day may not be healthy for patients or providers. Since most concierge and DPC providers receive a fixed amount of revenue for each client regardless of how often they visit, clinicians are not rewarded for maximizing patients' use of health care services. Instead, they're incentivized to get and keep their clients well. Smaller panels and less paperwork mean more provider/patient face time and, hopefully, less stress for everyone. In theory, improved overall health outcomes should also result from these models through better communication, proactive healthy living and more effective management of chronic conditions. Those are just two options that might threaten our existing patient-provider relationships, but that's not all older patients should be watching out for.

Wait! What? You've stopped taking Medicare?

We know Medicare and Medicaid reimbursement is considerably lower than that of commercial or private market health insurers for the same services and procedures. In addition, government health plans require compliance with mind-melting regulations. Health care providers can now reduce those burdens by choosing to limit the number of Medicare and/or Medicaid patients in their panel or refusing to take any. And some are.

CMS lists 26,000 doctors having officially opted out of Medicare, which would be a single digit percentage of all providers. However, these numbers don't reflect those who never enrolled in Medicare in the first place. A 2015 Kaiser Family Foundation survey showed 23 percent of primary care physicians either limiting or not accepting Medicare patients and 54 percent opting out or limiting Medicaid patients. More recently, the 2018 Physicians Foundation study puts those figures at 22 percent and 32 percent, respectively. In 2019, the Medicaid and CHIP Payment and Access Commission (MACPAC) put opt-out rates at 15 percent for Medicare and 29 percent for Medicaid.[286] (As for dental health care, 35 states provide limited adult dental benefits, but 38.5 percent of children receive dental care through Medicaid or the federal Children's Health Insurance Program (CHIP). Only 43 percent of dentists participate.[287])

As consumers, we should recognize our clinicians may one day decide to have fewer patients, to refuse some or all health insurance, to reduce hours to part-time or to retire early. Who can blame them? Although previous generations of doctors had stress, today's providers have something their predecessors never had: the option to consider the *business* of medicine as distinct from the *practice* of medicine. Innovations such as concierge and direct primary care models reduce the role of payers/insurers and return some or all decision-making power to the patient-provider team. After a closer look, we may find it's also in our best interests as health care consumers to embrace those concepts. Anyway, we know for sure that when providers and patients row in different directions, we get nowhere. Very shortly, I'm going to focus on action steps to preserve your rights to informed consent, autonomy and safety. Before that, however, let's see how Americans' lack of health literacy, the final element of the perfect storm, has been addressed by policy makers and stakeholders until now.

CHAPTER NINE

Lessons in how *not* to raise health literacy

Although health literacy, the third element of the perfect storm, is the reflection of an individual's decision-making skills, it is wholly dependent on the system at large to respect patient autonomy, to make options available and to provide vital information. Are policy makers and stakeholders doing all they can to help us be engaged, autonomous and safe health care consumers?

Working to address Americans' lack of health literacy is our one remaining opportunity to ready for the approaching storm. The level of health literacy you're able and willing to practice directly influences how you manage resources, preventive care, healthy living, medications, caregiving, shared decision making, chronic illness, handoffs, emergencies and the end of life. You name it—if a decision about health care has to be made, it is better made with health literacy on your side. Whatever resources end up being plentiful or scarce as we go forward, being health literate will make the highest and most efficient use of them. As importantly, health literacy preserves a patient's rights to informed consent, autonomy and safety.

To refresh your memory, health literacy is *not* functional literacy, which is being able to read, write or speak the local language. It is not knowing everything about a specific medical condition. It is not being able to perform math calculations. And it is not pronouncing medical terms properly—or knowing what they mean without first asking. Instead, being health literate might be seeking guidance on how to manage chronic pain; exploring all available treatment options for a life-limiting diagnosis; knowing when to get a second opinion; insisting on clear, unambiguous and written aftercare instructions before you leave the hospital; or having a list of questions to ask during your annual checkup (okay, being health literate is first making that appointment).

How can we tell if someone is health literate?

The long-standing definition of health literacy is *Recognizing when, how and where to access, process and understand basic health information and services needed to make informed decisions concerning medical treatment and care.* It's been around for well over two decades and is accepted worldwide. This well-established view of health literacy respects each patient's autonomous right to make informed choices, while recognizing it takes an acquired set of information-gathering and decision-making skills to preserve that right. This definition makes sense. Informed decision making has to be preceded by understanding.

Let me ask you a question. Would you agree that if you're confronted with a health care situation and the doctor clearly and fully explains available options and verifies your understanding, this patient-provider process would increase the chances you'll make an informed choice? Of course, because the provider's respect for your autonomy and right to shared decision making partnered with your engagement makes for better health outcomes. Congratulations, you understand what it takes to be health literate. The simple answer to the question *How can we tell if someone is health literate?* is *By asking*. However, you and I both know researchers seldom take the shortest route to anywhere.

Once health literacy became recognized as a measurable concept, people got into the business of measuring it. They're still at it. These are just some of the tools they've developed: Health Literacy Assessment Using Talking Touchscreen Technology (Health LiTT), Newest Vital Sign (NVS), Rapid Estimate of Adult Literacy in Medicine (REALM), REALM Short Form (REALM-SF), Test of Functional Health Literacy in Adults (TOFHLA), Cancer Health Literacy Test (CHLT-30), Health Literacy Questionnaire (HLQ), Information and Support for Health Actions Questionnaire (ISHA-Q), Behavioral Risk Factor Surveillance System (BRFSS/HL), Brief Health Literacy Screen (BHLS), Single Item Literacy Screener (SILS) and Health Literacy Skills Instrument (HLSI). These tests use a variety of models, from calculating an allowable portion of ice cream using a "nutrition facts" food label to reading a list of medical terms without stumbling. There's even a brief-and-to-the-point one-question health literacy test: *How often do you need to have someone help you when you read instructions, pamphlets or other written material from your doctor or pharmacy?* (A hint: Knowing when to ask for assistance is not seen as a good thing . . .) Until recently, that was my favorite. Not any more: "*Which human sense is the least studied of the five basic senses?*"[288] Now, why would anyone know such a thing, and if one did, how would knowing that increase the chances of making informed health care decisions? Good grief.

I'm not an academic, but I do recall from earning a degree in psychology that there are two prongs of research: *validity* (whether the test measures what it's meant to measure) and *reliability* (the consistency of the measurements). So I'm suspect of tools that infer a lack of health literacy because someone knows when they should ask a question or seek help. Really, have these people ever read a prescription Medication Guide? Other researchers choose more expeditious methods. The University of North Carolina at Chapel Hill developed a computer model revealing areas of limited health literacy down to the census block containing 600 to 3,000 people. Their predictive model "*estimates the mean health literacy of individuals living in each census block group*" by simply analyzing residents' gender, age, race, language, income, education, marital status and how long they've been in the country.[289] That is alarming on so many levels.

Admittedly, it isn't relevant whether or not I'm convinced any of those health literacy measuring tools are valid and/or reliable. The researchers who develop them believe they are, and to quote the Centers for Disease Control and Prevention," *The Federal government supports health literacy research!*"[290] Of *that* there is no doubt.

What we now know about health literacy

There have been more than 6,000 studies and publications featuring health literacy since 1991,[291] with an additional ten to 20 materializing each week. I subscribe to business guru Peter Drucker's famous quote, *If you can't measure it, you can't improve it,* but come on. Assuming studies are done to either confirm a theory or tell us something we didn't already know, what have we learned?

First, we know we need more research, as stated in every study—*every* one. In the Institute of Medicine's 2004 *Health Literacy – a Prescription to End Confusion*, 20 of the 21 recommendations for achieving a vision of health literacy in America were to conduct further research.[292] In 2016, more than 63 million Americans were surveyed on how easy it is to access and understand health care information. When 43 percent responded they found it "*very easy*," the researchers concluded the respondents' self-reported proficiency was grossly overstated. Once they determined we're not even health literate enough to know we're not health literate, they threw out the results and made ten recommendations for more research.[293]

The second most common finding of health literacy research is that providers should dumb down written and verbal communication to meet patients' diminished capacity to understand, you know, due to their lack of health literacy. Suggestions include using words of no more than two syllables, not providing too much information to patients and avoiding medical terminology. Specifically, health care professionals are encouraged to keep everything at a sixth grade reading level or below. One of the more popular suggestions, certainly among my followers and friends, has been for clinicians to explain medical issues in "*language that you might use when talking to your grandmother.*"[294] Clearly, they haven't dialogued recently with any of the grandmothers I know.

There's a ton of research on the "dumbing down" theory of health literacy alone. How is it being applied? Here's an example hot off the press: In the midst of the pandemic, Dartmouth did a study to learn whether COVID-19 information for the public was meeting recommended readability standards. They reviewed 137 COVID-19-related public health and government web pages and all were found in violation of warnings from the CDC, the American Medical Association and HHS's National Institutes of Health to keep medical information at the down low reading level.[295] Okay, but if the premise is valid, it might have been more constructive to use those findings in a practical way. Say, by applying the same readability standards to Dartmouth's own COVID-19 public information website, which I found is written at *five to seven grades above* those recommended readability standards for health care consumers.

What you and I haven't learned the hard way about the potential harm from bad or no communication, we've observed and heard from friends and family. Most of us don't need a college research institute to tell us we're not the effective health care advocates we'd like to be, for ourselves or on behalf of others. Over the past 20 years, I have also discovered quite a bit about consumers' willingness and ability to be health literate. Granted, my inferences come not from scientific studies but from hearing people talk about their willingness and ability to be health literate. My conclusion? The whole dumbing down theory is bogus. With few exceptions for identifiable capacity issues, every adult who wants to be more engaged and empowered can make fully informed and well-considered health care decisions—once their right to do so is acknowledged and they have access to practical health literacy tools. Since the one element of the perfect storm over which we have a large measure of control is our individual and collective levels of health literacy, it's in our best interests to ask: *Is all this health literacy research being used to make our health care journeys more health literate?*

They have a plan, just not for us

A few years after the U.S. Department of Education released its landmark findings about Americans' lack of health literacy, HHS began formulating multiple strategies to address those deficiencies.[296] What followed was its 2010 *National Action Plan to Improve Health Literacy.* The stated vision was to provide access to health information, deliver person-centered health information and services and support lifelong learning and skills to promote good health. It sounds good for us but it really isn't. The Introduction to the *Action Plan* clearly states its target audience is health care professionals, public and private sector organizations, communities and policy makers—not health care consumers, as one might assume from reading that mission statement.[297] In this plan to raise Americans' health literacy, what's missing is any goal supporting the rightful decision makers: patients and their advocates.

The same can be said for materials developed by HHS to supplement that 2010 *Action Plan*, such as the *Health Literacy Care Model* and *Health Literacy Online – A Guide for Simplifying the User Experience.*[298] These campaigns illustrate policy makers' perplexing approach to health literacy: First, they conclude the difficulty stems entirely from the patient's side. Then they disregard any solutions that might make patients more health literate decision makers.

Health literacy was also a named objective in the *Healthy People 2010* and *Healthy People 2020* initiatives from HHS, more do-nothing strategies for assisting patients to master health literacy fundamentals, such as shared decision making and chronic care management. Instead, HHS initiatives measure Americans' progress in achieving health literacy by the number of health care-related websites and the census of those with broadband internet access.[299] Whatever the objectives du jour may be, we've seen the overall success of the *Healthy People* series. Besides their ineffectual redundancy, these programs fail to advance any goals associated with the achievement of health literacy.

Sadly, little benefit from three decades of health literacy research has trickled down to those who could really use the decision making and care management support, patients and their advocates. With few exceptions, organizational efforts to improve health literacy are directed at medicine's mega health systems and providers, rather than those whose rights are threatened and most directly impacted by bad or deficient medical decisions. Even with the purported goal of improved health literacy, programs are intended not to support patient autonomy but to bring down costs, improve value and, in some cases, meet payers' quality control requirements.[300]

There are no less than ten subagencies under HHS dedicated to *the science and practice of health literacy improvement.*[301] The mission statements of the federal programs leading these efforts speak for themselves. Who is the intended audience for HHS's official home of health literacy, the Office of Disease Prevention and Health Promotion (ODPHP)? *Health professionals.* At the Agency for Healthcare Research and Quality (AHRQ), where the goal is to make sure patient safety research findings are understood and used? *Health care professionals and delivery organizations.* At the Centers for Disease Control and Prevention (CDC)? *Health communicators, public health professionals and community leaders.*[302] It's like solving the problem of functional illiteracy in America's schools by hoping to make teachers better readers.

As for other attempts to help patients improve decision making, the CDC proudly lists all state and local collaborations and academic, government and nonprofit organizations working toward those goals. Scrutinizing those 22 (of a potential 50) states' programs supporting health literacy efforts, we find nine are actually websites selling professional services to providers; eight sites either don't exist, aren't about health literacy or have not been updated for years; and four contain nothing more than hyperlinks to other government websites. Hats off to Ohio, shown as offering legitimate health literacy resources to its residents. Worth mention is the state university that misspelled *literacy* on its website.[303]

You know those times when no matter how hard someone tries, they still miss the target? This isn't that. In viewing the consistent failure of policy makers and stakeholders to help Americans be better health care decision makers and care managers, missing the target is no surprise when they consistently and intentionally aim in the wrong direction. Now, if it's research, websites, conferences, plain language consultants or smartphone apps you're looking for, they've got you covered. As just one example, HHS's Agency for Healthcare Research and Quality awarded $250,000 in prize money in 2018 for the development of a health care smartphone app. Plucky of them, when there are already more than 300,000 commercially-produced apps available for download—with another 200 being added daily.[304] I receive a barrage of e-mails everyday with the latest health care-related research and news. I got pretty excited when I saw a newspaper article bragging on a state's efforts to improve health literacy. Red herring. They've formed a coalition with the goal of having conferences, doing research, writing grants and forming a statewide collaborative. I'm not seeing how any of that assists the state's residents in becoming better medical decision makers.

The endgame of informed health care decision making is to achieve the best health outcomes for patients, considering their autonomous circumstances and preferences. It requires them to be engaged and health literate members of a care team. That can't happen as long as the patient's role is absent from strategies to improve health literacy. Likewise, measuring, analyzing and evaluating health literacy is not the same as putting information-gathering and decision-making tools into the hands of patients and advocates and clinicians. Frankly, I wouldn't know how to write a 175-page health literacy toolkit for primary care providers and never touch on shared decision making. Nor could I approach the subject of care management without encouraging active patient participation. Yet you will find health literacy training materials from government agencies and stakeholders manage to do both, very well.[305]

It's déjà vu all over again

Turns out we've seen this movie before, so we know how it ends. When lawmakers decided health care advance directives would resolve the issue of medical decision making once and for all, Congress passed the 1990 *Patient Self-Determination Act* (PSDA), still in effect. It requires health care providers to ask all patients if they have a Durable Power of Attorney for Health Care and/or a Living Will, to explain the right to have them and to promise not to discriminate on the basis of whether they do. The PSDA also mandates Advance Care Planning education for the public and for health care professionals. Naturally, that last part never really took off, but it's fair to say the PSDA is responsible for the dramatic increase in the proportion of Americans with advance directives. Over the past 30 years, it's gone from 15 to 20 percent of adults to today's mind-blowing rate of 26 to 29 percent.[306] The story at the beginning of this book about the emergency department patient is just one example of the pervasive ignorance that continues to surround advance directives. All of which goes to show you what three decades of government dedication to public health care education can accomplish.

In the interest of partisan parity, health literacy initiatives have been embedded in the mission of HHS (fka the U.S. Department of Health, Education and Welfare) throughout eight presidential administrations and more sessions of Congress than anyone cares to think about. There's plenty of attribution for both sides of the aisle. The stated goals of every proposed health literacy action plan have been safety, comprehensive health care and more accessible resources. Over the decades, America's health care leaders have unswervingly failed to achieve anything even remotely close to those objectives. While it is not researchers' role to effect change in the system, it most definitely *is* the job of policy makers and bureaucrats to implement relevant findings for the benefit of those who can use the information—and have probably paid for the studies to be done. In fact, it's the verbatim mission statement of one such federal bureau, the Agency for Healthcare Research and Quality (AHRQ): *To produce evidence to make health care safer, higher quality, more accessible, equitable, and affordable, and to work within the U.S. Department of Health and Human Services and with other partners to make sure that the evidence is understood and used.*[307] With that in mind, what are policy makers now working on to improve health literacy in America?

Surgical removal of the patient from decision making

The latest development in the advancement of health literate decision making and care management is not entirely unexpected. With every one of these credited to HHS, the definition of health literacy has been evolving since its first use in 1974:

- *The "patients merit self-advocacy" approach:* Health literacy is the degree to which individuals have the capacity to obtain, process, and understand basic health information needed to make appropriate health decisions[308] to
- *The "dumbing down to the patient's level" approach:* Health literacy occurs when health information and services created for the public match with people's capacity to find, understand, and use them[309] to
- *The "our work here is done" approach:* Health literacy occurs when a society provides accurate health information and services people can easily find, understand, and use to inform their decisions and actions.[310]

I'm not entirely sure what that third definition even means. It sure sounds like HHS is saying health literacy is achieved once health care info and services are available, whether or not consumers access, understand and use them to become informed and engaged decision makers. This creative approach is like suggesting someone is functionally literate because the library down the block has been stocked with books.

(I get I'm probably the only health literacy geek in the room right now, but I promise this is a revealing narrative.) The HHS staff who were fine-tuning *Healthy People 2030* in 2019 filed a formal notice seeking public comment on their intent to officially adopt that third definition of *health literacy*. Granted, implementing this view of health literacy would certainly be a break for those who measure it. Forget asking individuals about their understanding of the health care decision making process. A population's level of health literacy equates to the number of consumers with broadband internet access, the mounting assortment of health care-related websites and smartphone apps or perhaps a clinic's volume of large-print brochures. Wait a minute—this sounds strangely familiar and explains a lot. The *Healthy People* initiatives have been measuring gains in health literacy using those exact metrics for decades. On the other hand, I have to wonder what happens to the nearly 300 health literacy projects currently being funded by the NIH if a whole new definition is adopted. Not to mention the $67 million in research underway through the Patient-Centered Outcomes Research Institute (PCORI). I'm no academic scientist, but it seems if there's a seismic shift in the basic meaning of the subject being studied, the research would be impacted.[311] Anyway, never mind. It's all moot.

HHS got no shortage of public responses to its proposed definition change in 2019 and most observers were just as confused as I.[312] Not a problem, because soon after, they ditched that idea and instead approved this new *two-part definition* of health literacy, without the bother of any public input:

- *Personal health literacy* is the degree to which individuals have the ability to find, understand, and use information and services to inform health-related decisions and actions for themselves and others.
- *Organizational health literacy* is the degree to which organizations equitably enable individuals to find, understand, and use information and services to inform health-related decisions and actions for themselves and others.[313]

I freely admit I don't get it. How does anything other than a human achieve health literacy? Unless they're talking about *artificial health literacy*, and maybe they are . . . Here's where the whole thing truly becomes a riddle, wrapped in a mystery. The initial draft of *Healthy People 2030* contained a ten-year objective to increase Americans' health literacy, and why wouldn't it? Health literacy was previously included in both *Healthy People 2010* and *Healthy People 2020*; it's a natural prerequisite for people to be healthy. Nevertheless, after all the pomp, circumstance, man hours and expense invested in altering the definition, *health literacy* was summarily dropped as an objective from *Healthy People 2030* just prior to its launch in late 2020. Here's the explanation from HHS: "*This objective* [health literacy] *has research status, meaning it is a high-priority public health issue that doesn't yet have evidence-based interventions developed to address it. It may or may not have reliable baseline data available.*"

Let me get this straight and you along with me: After 30 years of research and more than 6,000 studies, health literacy has not risen above the level of "*research status*" at HHS?[314] Meanwhile, the HHS subagency in charge of the *Healthy People* initiatives, the Office of Disease Prevention and Health Promotion, continues to boast of how the updated definition of *health literacy* is helping to achieve the goals of *Healthy People 2030.* Apparently, they've forgotten they deleted *health literacy* from the initiative before its launch. A riddle wrapped in a mystery inside an enigma.[315] Consequently, there are now no less than four different definitions of *health literacy* in use throughout the subagencies of HHS. Naturally, designing research to measure how an *organization* can be health literate is in full swing. These people are exhausting.

So, there you are. It is official: Assisting health care's end users to learn and apply health literate decision making and care management is not something our policy makers aspire to. Just when the Boomers could seriously use some help in managing complex and chronic medical conditions, those best positioned as health literacy's primary change agents have concluded we are not educable. If we are, it's not their job to do it. And if it is, they choose not to. These missteps and pointless administrative maneuvers say more than I ever could about the bureaucratic value placed on patients' rights to informed consent. Sigh.

Post-surgery recovery

Why should you and I even care which definition of health literacy is being adopted and promoted by federal agencies? Practically speaking, when the doctor delivers an unexpected diagnosis and a treatment decision needs to be made *pronto*, the only relevant measure of *health literacy* is whether you have the decision-making fundamentals it takes to be a confident and empowered advocate. Will you know when to insist on a board-certified specialist, to recognize if a loved one needs caregiving assistance or how to manage medications?

The reason we should care is because words matter, especially when they drive health care policy. This comes down to the respect being given to our role as patients in deciding whether and how health care is delivered. At the end of the day, an institutional mindset ends up embedded in legislation, agency mission statements and strategic plans. It governs funding for research, providers' reimbursement for services and how many people get to become doctors. It determines the availability of well baby clinics, health screenings for seniors and hospice care appropriations. Messing with any of those health care components negatively impacts the affordability of and access to health care and, ultimately, whether we achieve the best possible health outcomes.

Raise your hand if you're aware of a government-sponsored program to assist health care consumers in becoming more engaged and empowered. Or you've heard a public service announcement about how patients can be safer. Or witnessed a press conference on the looming health care labor shortages. No, me neither. In a way, it's a relief to finally appreciate and acknowledge where we stand. Policy makers' failure to help consumers be the best possible advocates for themselves and others solidifies once and for all that *we are on our own*. It is indisputably up to each one of us to preserve decision-making rights, protect patient autonomy and remain as safe as possible while mucking our way through the health care system.

Chapters Eleven through Sixteen contain guidance for doing all that. You'll learn that health literacy essentials are the information-gathering and decision-making skills you can use to move toward accessible, appropriate and safe health care. Forget all the bureaucratic posturing, because very little of it is aimed at preserving patient autonomy. You are the sole determinant of whether you achieve health literacy and then apply its fundamentals to be an informed decision maker. As you are about to learn, if you are willing, you are able. *You've got this*.

PART THREE

Strategies for self-preservation

CHAPTER TEN

Aim to be at the table, not on the menu

Ever board a plane on a dark, dreary day and then climb atop the clouds? Your attitude is immediately improved. It's like magic. Likewise, as health care crises materialize in your life, as they are apt to do, you will optimize your options and outcomes if you will learn to rise above the perfect storm.

An endless source of joy and disappointment

If health care as it now exists in America were a block-buster movie, the trailer might sound something like this (cue deep-voiced narrator):

Coming soon, in a health care system where anything can happen . . .

An approaching disaster so vast only a bureaucrat could fail to see it . . .

The masters of suspense and horror now bring you . . .

We've witnessed decades of what passes for policy makers' leadership in anticipating and overcoming inevitable obstacles to health care access and safety, as evidenced by their boundless commitment to research, proposals, action plans, checklists, committees, white papers, advisory boards, mnemonics, collaboratives, toolkits and strategic alliances. Judge for yourself, but I'm ready to say I don't think we can depend on them as partners—let alone as leaders—in preparing for the approaching perfect storm of health care. Now, having acknowledged that, we can plan accordingly.

The preceding chapters were brutal. I didn't relish spending so many pages on what lies under the rocks, but there was no other way for you to fully appreciate what's coming. Let's be honest, it's simply not in our collective DNA to focus on stuff not an immediate threat to our well-being. Nevertheless, it's time to shift the mode from problem to solution, which means learning all we can about self-preservation in the midst of a wholly foreseeable perfect storm. Health care stakeholders and policy makers are preparing for the approaching crisis much as they've readied for every other major phase in the Boomers' lives: by first spotting it in the rearview mirror. Take, for instance, those outdated and inexplicable workforce projections from HHS/HRSA. If they end up being wrong—which rational people would bet they are—the bureaucratic equivalent of "*Our bad*" will be of little solace to the patient who dies waiting for EMTs.

You may be thinking, *Why haven't I heard about all this before?* Or you may be questioning the veracity of what you've read so far. Actually, many have been talking about this for a very long time, including a plethora of Surgeons General beginning in the 1970s. Yes, way back when Boomers were in their 20s and 30s, soothsayers were already predicting they would one day be in their 60s and 70s. You've seen the evidence of this demographic tsunami for yourself. In addition to the personal challenges of aging and chronic illness, there are systemic hazards in the path leading to our best possible health outcomes, and you have a good idea of what they are. Whether or not health care's institutional change agents are willing or equipped to properly meet these imminent obstacles, our commitment to be prepared as health care consumers must not waiver.

Danger, Will Robinson!

Up until now, we have blindly relied on "the system" to anticipate and overcome every potential barrier to access, to light the way on our health care journeys. What we learned when COVID-19 hit was that while we thought "they" had potential obstacles and disasters all sussed out, they didn't. That was a costly and valuable lesson, but even when we're not facing a pandemic, there are obvious clear and present dangers for us as health care consumers. Among them are demographic realities, competition for access, preventable medical errors and time constraints that thwart shared decision making. But before pointing fingers, we should recognize our own role in failing to have the best possible health outcomes, and that includes the willful ignorance of our rights as patients. We don't get to disrespect ourselves, then complain about getting no respect.

This is where we've set the health care bar for a very long time, because that's just who we are:

- I want to make lifestyle choices without regard to the impact on my health.
- I want a pill to relieve all symptoms.
- I want every disease to have a cure.
- I want comprehensive health care to be reasonably priced—better yet, free.
- And I want health care when I need it and where I am.

Along with the right to give consent comes the responsibility to be fully informed in medical decision making—the polar opposite of ignoring common sense, making bad choices, refusing to be engaged in care management and not reaching our full potential as health care advocates. Prioritizing self-preservation is pragmatic and fundamental to being a valued health care team member, and patient activation begins when you become aware of your rights and act responsibly to preserve them. If the bloated health care system fails to acknowledge and address known risks, then it is in our best interests to have the skills and awareness needed to avoid them when possible.

Going with wishful thinking or regret?

Although we can certainly learn from past mistakes, there is no future in setting our sights anywhere but on the road ahead as we work to prepare for this perfect storm's arrival. As for changing the course of demographics, fuggedaboutit. It's equally beyond our scope as consumers to address health care labor and financial shortages, if that's even possible. But ask me if there's still time for someone to become an empowered and activated health care consumer and I'd say *absolutely*. While it is true that of all the chess pieces, the pawn has the fewest options for movement, the good news is *the pawn can only move forward.*

Wishful thinking is when you say, *If only we had known what was going to happen, we would have made a different decision.* That comes from failing to be intuitive and I can't help you there. On the other hand, *regret* is looking back and thinking, *If we had really understood the situation, we would have made a different decision.* Regret comes not from making a choice that turned out to be wrong, but from making a decision that was erroneous from the get-go because it lacked foundation. Using the tools and processes of health literacy to be fully informed is something we *can* work toward.

At this time and place in history, we are constantly reminded of possible threats to our safety. Not having access to appropriate and competent health care is one of them. For most perils, the potential for any single person to make a difference is limited. Exercising the absolute power of informed decision making in the management of your health care is the welcome exception but only if you claim your authority. In the game of health care, you'll want to be within arm's reach of a chair when the music stops.

The time for action has come

I am of the opinion we should begin to demand what is ours for the taking: the autonomous right to be treated with respect as we cope with acute conditions, chronic disease and aging. Throughout the remainder of this book, you will learn strategies to help you become the engaged health care decision maker you must be to take your rightful place in line for timely and appropriate health care. There's no reason we should settle for less. We do so at our own peril.

Who do I think I'm talking to? Well, anyone who will listen, but I do have one message just for the benefit of a younger cohort. "*OK Boomer*" is a slang term some Millennials have used to voice their opinion of what they consider stereotypical Boomer behaviors—usually in a mocking tone. First, not all Boomers are alike, a lesson we've more than learned in the recent past. Second, I'm statistically certain 99 percent of Boomers won't be around to help pay for the care Millennials will need in their golden years. Perhaps once the Millennials figure out America's age thing doesn't level off until 2060, they might be more on board to link arms with Boomers on this mission of patient autonomy and safety. I'm just saying, we'd be glad to have them on our side.

For the past 90 pages, I've covered how we got to where we now find ourselves. Identifying the problem is important, even crucial, but awareness is of little value unless it's followed by action steps moving us closer to self-preservation. *Praemonitus, praemunitus. Forewarned is forearmed.* Otherwise, we're stuck where many have been for decades, doing research. It has helped very little. Once we acknowledge there may not be adequate resources for everyone, as advocates for ourselves and others, our objective must be to be treated with respect and compassion. But, first and foremost, to be treated. That means doing whatever it takes to access timely and safe health care, no matter what our autonomous circumstances may be.

Some might say the outlook is dismal, so what's the point? I reject that premise. I have boundless respect for the innate capacity of health care consumers to be fully engaged with even just a little help. There are ways to surround yourself with competent, appropriate and well-informed health care, and we'll explore them in the coming chapters. Fair warning: Being engaged, empowered, autonomous and safe is not without its obligations, and this may be your last opportunity to remain in the land of blissful ignorance. It's time to aim for self-preservation, in spite of America's perfect storm of health care: *Patient or pawn?*

CHAPTER ELEVEN

Health Literacy: The secret ingredient

To have any hope of preserving rights to informed consent, autonomy and safety while achieving the best health outcomes, you'll need a process for engaged and empowered decision making. It's the secret to remaining visible. This skill set known as health literacy is the foundation of self-preservation.

Informed advocacy is Job One

Before we go any further, let's get something clear. Maybe the government's top health care policy makers and leaders haven't budged beyond "*research status*" and don't yet know enough about health literacy to grasp its significance and move forward—but not you and me. Not only can we clearly recognize the struggles that nearly always precede bad decision making, we're eager and ready to overcome them. Let's get to the business of becoming the empowered patients we deserve and are destined to be.

Everyone's familiar with the concept of IQ, *intelligence quotient*, which is defined as the ability to acquire and then apply knowledge and skills. Similarly, a person's *health literacy*—we'll just call it HQ—is recognizing when, how and where to access, process and understand the basic health information and services needed to make informed choices. And, for the record, there is no evidence of a direct correlation between IQ and HQ. None.

When people aren't health literate and lack the skills and tools to effectively manage health care, they don't live as long or as well. We also know when health care professionals and patients do implement health literate practices, hospital readmissions are reduced; health care costs are dramatically cut; and we add to the quality, quantity and safety of patients' lives. If estimates are accurate, medical errors are the third leading cause of death in America. And if true, it's also scandalous, since recommended strategies for preventing almost all medical mistakes are identical to the fundamentals of health literacy.

HQ is not so different from IQ. Just as IQ isn't possessing specific knowledge, achieving health literacy isn't being a medical expert, it's a process for information gathering in preparation for informed decision making. Here's an example of the opposite of being health literate. It seems everyone knows someone with rotator cuff issues, so we throw the medical term around like we know what we're talking about. *Sounds like it could be the rotator cuff. I'll bet it's his rotator cuff. Yeah, Dr. Soandso fixed my neighbor's rotator cuff.* Let me tell you, I learned the meaning of "rotator cuff" when I managed to severely tear mine. I could have avoided that injury if I had explored the dangers inherent in lifting heavy objects or had bothered to learn even a little about the physiology of raising my arm or had relied on a source of medical knowledge other than jibber-jabber over appetizers. Regrettably, I didn't know what I didn't know about the care and preservation of rotator cuffs, which turned out to be a lot. And when I was finally forced to seek medical expertise, a lack of health literate communication between my doctor and me very nearly cost me the use of my arm.

Being health literate is recognizing there's real value in preventive care. It's asking for a moment to collect your thoughts when you can't grasp what the doctor's telling you. It's understanding the immeasurable value of having someone along during important consultations. It's having a backup plan for caregiving in the event of an unexpected crisis, say, a pandemic. And it's doing everything in your power to avoid the hazards of medical errors, as an advocate for yourself or for someone else.

People with accurate information—and enough of it—make better decisions and live longer. Weird, right? Moreover, when we throw autonomy into the decision-making mix, we find the informed and autonomous choice for one patient may be very different than for the guy in the next bed. Indeed, that is the ultimate goal of health literate decision making: To achieve the best health outcomes for the person whose health and well-being hang in the balance.

Strategies for self-preservation / Health literacy

Chapter Nine covered what has previously passed as policy makers' attempts to raise Americans' health literacy. Instead of concentrating on how to pronounce medical terms or calculate allowable calories in a dish of ice cream (who really cares?), you and I will focus on action steps intended to move you toward being a more empowered patient. Health literacy has three basic building blocks and they apply in every health care situation:

A. *Identify and access reliable health literacy resources.*

B. *Practice shared decision making.*

C. *Take documentation action steps.*[316]

Being health literate means practicing informed, engaged and empowered health care decision making and implementing these ten fundamentals of health literacy:

#10 Reliable health care information Whether checking out a symptom or seeking a second opinion, find and stick with comprehensive, current and independently verifiable sources. That applies to getting recommendations for a provider, looking for online information, making a critical medical decision or managing a chronic condition.

And, FYI, Internet chat rooms are nothing more than cyber soap boxes for all manner of anonymous persons, including angry people in jammies.

#9 Health care advocacy First and foremost, let's begin with the premise that each one of us *must* self-advocate, at all times knowing and preserving rights to informed consent, autonomy and safety. The only thing more ill-advised than leaving the management of one's health care to chance would be leaving it to unnamed others. The health care proxy and guardian are preplanned backups in case of temporary or permanent incapacity. Just do it.

#8 Assembling a health care team The choice of providers—and many people have more than one—greatly influences whether someone has the best possible health outcomes. Choose with care, considering the patient's unique needs and the provider's unique talents. Never be afraid to ask a health care professional, "*Who would you recommend for yourself or a family member?*" An estimated one quarter to one half of American adults do not have a primary care provider. When a health care need arises is not the time to start looking for the most qualified leader of your health care team. Assuming you're able to get an appointment in a pinch, a new doctor won't know you, not even a little. Empowered patients are proactive patients.

#7 Caregiving Whether it's daily meal delivery, assistance with medications or full-time residential care, the need for appropriate, competent and compassionate caregiving in the midst of labor shortages requires planning. Openly and honestly evaluate present and potential needs and verify available resources—you may need to get on a waiting list or start making adjustments. Remember to care for the caregiver.

#6 Preventive care Preventive care is treatment meant to either stop a medical condition from occurring or discover an otherwise hidden issue. Timely tests and vaccinations can be lifesaving, so learn what's appropriate for your gender, age, ethnicity, existing conditions and family history. Be part of the population who sees a doctor at least once a year. It's also a great opportunity to cultivate that patient-provider relationship.

#5 Medication and polypharmacy With six billion prescriptions filled in America each year, it's no wonder a doctor opined that any new symptom should be assumed to be drug-related until proven otherwise. This topic got its own chapter (Fifteen).

#4 Urgent care versus Emergency care Health literacy embraces being mindful of symptoms, knowing when and where to turn for expertise (human or cyber) and planning to take appropriate steps if the need arises. Knowing the difference between *emergency care* and *urgent care* is crucial, much like the difference between lightning and a lightning bug.[317] It includes mastering your role as the advocate in an emergency and, sorry, but that takes preparation.

#3 Palliative care and hospice care There has always been confusion surrounding these two specialties. Palliative care, also known as comfort care, is appropriate to alleviate the symptoms of any disease or the side effects of treatment. Anyone managing a chronic condition or being treated for an acute or serious medical issue may benefit. Hospice is palliative care reserved for the end of life. And both also address the emotional, spiritual, medical and practical needs of the patient's concerned persons. Recognizing when you should pursue these distinct specialties is key to making the most of available resources. Life is measured in quality as well as quantity.

#2 Documentation action steps This is the part most people don't want to think about or discuss. May I suggest it's a bit disingenuous to expect a health care professional to give autonomous and appropriate health care treatment to a stranger, with no knowledge of the patient's history, medications, allergies, wishes for care, et cetera? Creating an accessible record of your medications, medical history, medical devices, advance directives and contacts takes a few hours. A few life-altering hours.

[drum roll]

#1 Shared decision making If these ten fundamentals are the foundation of health literacy, this is the cornerstone. Shared decision making involves a provider being fully aware of the patient's medical and personal stories *and* a health care decision maker being fully informed of treatment options. It's been around since 1982, and the steps are few and simple:

1. The health care issue requiring a decision is fully summarized.
2. The patient's story and values are shared, including personal and treatment goals.
3. The provider explains all available care options, risks and benefits.
4. Choices are fully discussed and considered by all concerned parties.
5. Fully informed consent is given by either the patient or substitute decision maker.

Part of the shared decision making process is seeking a second opinion when either the diagnosis or proposed treatment is life-threatening or uncertain or the proposed treatment is experimental. Or when something just doesn't feel right.

Sometimes being health literate is as simple as knowing when to speak up. Like when you ask about the prognosis for an elderly patient and the doctor's response is, "*Well, after all, he is 93.*" That would be a good time to speak up, perhaps to ask, *At exactly what age should someone stop expecting the best health outcomes, doctor?* And, by the way, also a good time to start looking for a new provider.

Being aware of, encouraging and practicing the fundamentals of health literacy is acknowledging and compensating for inevitable human frailties and having practical methods to sidestep them. But before you can be heard, you must first be seen.

CHAPTER TWELVE

Try really hard not to be invisible

There are those who believe people really can make themselves invisible. Not saying that talent wouldn't come in handy at times, but this chapter focuses on Webster's traditional definition: Being of such small size or unobtrusive quality as to be hardly noticeable. If you suffer from this condition while trying to access health care, your medical issue will quickly take on secondary importance.

Did you once have a doctor who served you for decades, maybe even brought you into this world? He was the only physician you saw, never rushed you during visits and looked you in the eye, undistracted by a laptop. Treatment and care decision making were easily managed because available options were limited or nowhere to be found. Do we long for those days? Sure, except the part about cancers going undetected until it was too late for treatment or the thousands who died before automatic external defibrillators came along.

For a variety of reasons, it's no longer so easy to maintain exclusive, long-term patient-provider relationships. To begin with, fewer than ten percent of deliveries are still performed by family physicians;[318] there's less time for patient-provider interaction; those with chronic conditions often see multiple specialists; and if hospitalized, we're most likely under the care of a stranger/hospitalist. Not least of all, if you make it through this decade, there's a one in three chance the doctor now serving you will retire before you expire. While the viability of the monogamous patient-provider relationship is in jeopardy, the patient's role in decision making was already being marginalized on both the individual and system levels. This is not good.

The two sides of the coin

The critical function of shared decision making in the tool box of health literacy is obvious, but let's back up and review the legal and ethical reasons behind its significance. Whether founded on constitutional grounds of privacy or due process, the *right of consent* means every person is entitled to give permission for a medical procedure before it begins or to stop a treatment already started, with few exceptions. In an emergency, the right to informed consent is briefly suspended for the sake of expedient lifesaving; and a guardian or a health care proxy can step in when someone lacks decision making capacity, either temporarily or permanently.

Informed consent is one part of the health care shared decision-making paradigm. The other side of the ethical tug of war plaguing lawmakers, judges, patients and providers for as long as anyone's been keeping track is the doctor's *duty to disclose.* Before fully informed consent can be granted, the physician has an obligation to disclose what's at stake, available treatment options, the goals of each and any known risks. Even when choices seem limited—or virtually nonexistent—the patient has a right to know the truth of the condition, realistic treatment objectives and foreseeable outcomes. It immediately begs the questions, *As a patient, how much information do I need to make a truly informed decision? And how much do* <u>*you*</u> *need? Or the next person?* In fact, the provider is charged with communicating all information concerning the health care situation at hand measured by what a reasonable person in that particular patient's position would consider material to decision making.[319] Hmm . . .

My surgeon recommended rotator cuff surgery to prevent me from doing further, and possibly irreparable, damage. I knew my goal was to maintain a certain quality of life, so once I understood available treatment options, I didn't need gobs of detail about the inherent risks because they were unavoidable if I wanted to proceed. In contrast, if the proposed procedure had been heart surgery, there would have been numerous and potentially life-altering risks to consider, the possibility of noninvasive therapies and many decisions to be made. That's when it's up to the physician to determine what a reasonable person—whatever that means—would consider *material* to decision making under those unique circumstances. Fair warning to my providers: Like most patients, my perspective is tangled up with my medical history, my lifestyle, my personal goals, my values, my tolerance for risk, my tolerance for pain (low) and my personality. So although the physician doesn't need to know *everything* about me, he does need to know *something*. Yeah, this conversation is going to take more than 19.9 minutes, doc.

There is absolutely no reason to think practitioners don't want to be the very best at what they do. Almost all acknowledge they could use more time and assistance in adequately managing their patients' care.[320] With nearly every health literacy tool focused exclusively on providers, you'd think there's plenty of support for them to learn and then guide their patients in shared decision making. Take a closer look:

- Even though we know practice makes better communicators and clinicians,[321] medical schools include only two to seven hours of instruction on shared decision making.[322]
- After training only 800 health care professionals in its SHARE decision-making protocol, HHS abandoned this two-year-old train-the-trainer project in 2016.[323]
- The same is true of the shared decision making pilot programs for Medicare and Medicaid created by CMS. Both were scuttled in February of 2018 before their launchings, without explanation.[324]

- Only half of surveyed doctors know Medicare pays for chronic care management, which provides oversight of patient decision making and compliance with treatment plans. Others choose not to offer this patient service because of the low reimbursement rate, complex coding and CMS paperwork burden.[325]

Nevertheless, to fulfill the duty of disclosure, the physician needs the willingness, skills and time to learn about the patient's background along with the medical condition at hand. Getting to know patients well enough to sense what it's like to be in their shoes is, admittedly, as much instinct as science, but it's the only way a patient can avoid being *hardly noticeable* in the decision making process.

As the pandemic's tendrils reached into every segment of American health care, there was no shortage of activists arguing for their approach to treatment and how to fund it. Take a wild guess who was without a voice and without a seat on the countless coronavirus advisory boards, round tables and consortiums across the nation. Yes, health care consumers. The change agents get points for consistency.

Not that we aren't all acquainted with those who prefer to remain oblivious in the management of their own health care. An astonishing number of them, really, and probably not among the readers of this book. Still, research shows most patients want far more information than is typically disclosed. Lousy communication is the biggest obstacle to fully effective shared decision making, creating a serious disconnect between what providers say and what patients hear and vice versa.[326] Now we just need to bring these two sides together.

Hey, remember me? The patient?

Autonomy. It's why you may be stunned by my health care decision, when it seems like such an obvious choice to me. Autonomy incorporates an individual's personal values and moral independence into decision making without any undue influence on the person's free will—and that's more than simply the absence of arm twisting. It's also undue influence when the holder of information is not sharing everything you should know. Free will is premised on having all the facts, and there it is: We've circled around and find ourselves back at *fully informed consent*. It's what makes shared decision making indistinguishable from autonomous decision making.

Let's just admit that for a very long time our failure to practice effective patient-provider communication has resulted in disregard for patient autonomy. Here are a few research examples:

- An overwhelming majority of patients have no idea their chemotherapy treatments are not curing their cancers, only 5 percent fully understand their medical condition and 38 percent have never discussed their prognosis or life expectancy with a doctor.[327] Patients missing key pieces of pertinent information cannot possibly be giving fully informed consent to autonomous treatment plans.

- Two thirds of patients arrive at surgery without signed consent forms and two thirds of spinal surgery medical malpractice claims are due to a failure to obtain informed consent by explaining risks and treatment options.[328] This needs no clarification.
- Less than half of patients with terminal brain cancer are asked about end-of-life wishes or resuscitation code preferences, and only one third of ICU patient conferences included end-of-life value considerations, such as spirituality.[329] Both demonstrate a disregard for autonomy and the right to make choices while able.
- Some health care professionals are still debating whether it's okay to lie to a patient.[330] For the record, it is not. *Benevolent deception,* which is intentional misleading or the omission of information to protect the patient, may have been an acceptable practice in the 1800s. This is not the 1800s.
- In spite of the proliferation of triggering mnemonics and simplified forms to ascertain and record patient wishes, end-of-life care preferences are ignored for 38 percent of dying patients, one fourth are unaware they have do-not-resuscitate orders in their chart and 40 percent don't understand their medical issue is terminal.[331]

We need not wonder if we have the right to decide whether to start a new prescription, to have a hip replaced or to refuse a feeding tube. We do, without question. (Getting an insurer to approve the procedure is a whole other issue.) No matter how little the media, public lawmakers and stakeholders understood about *Quinlan, Cruzan* and *Schiavo*, the right to consent has been settled law in the United States since the late 1800s.[332] And providers needn't get all prickly over the implications, because health literacy and autonomy don't exclude the health care professional from decision making and care management. Quite the contrary, shared decision making takes the patient-provider health care relationship from paternalism to partnership.

I must confess this discussion barely touches on reality for our most vulnerable populations, who are invisible by definition. I speak of those who are economically underprivileged, intellectually disabled, dealing with mental health issues, unbefriended or the *oldest old*, meaning those aged 85 and older. The truth is, they have a faint, if any, voice in their health care, which extends to the choice of provider, treatment plan, care preferences—you name it. They are pretty much unseen and unheard and possess virtually no prospects for altering that. How will the coming health care-related industry shortages impact the deference given to their autonomy? May I suggest that without major systemic improvements, not in a good way.

As consumers in today's complex health care environment, we must focus on 1) knowing and asserting our rights to full disclosure and consent; 2) insisting on our lawful and responsible role in shared decision making and care management; and

3) accessing all the reliable information we need before making health care decisions. Take note that to be successful, every one of those key elements is dependent on actions being taken by the patient and/or the patient's advocate.

The U.S. Constitution and all the statutes, court decisions, regulations and patient bills of rights are just pieces of paper until you put their principles into action. Rejecting the paternalistic model of medical decision making is the first step in preserving your rights as a patient. But it's a meaningless gesture without the corresponding commitment to be an engaged and proactive health care advocate. If you don't want others to have absolute control over your health care and you fail to step up to the task yourself, your health care destiny is left flapping in the wind.

Strategies for self-preservation / Being visible

In health care situations from the mundane to the life-threatening, you simply cannot take your eye off the ball. The list below doesn't cover all the contingencies—that's an impossibility. These are representative examples to help you appreciate the variety of circumstances that can impact whether you receive appropriate and competent health care and ultimately have the best possible health outcomes.

- When you know something just doesn't seem right, say so and do not accept "*Don't worry about it*" as a response. Be respectful but firm. Do not back down.
- Practice this phrase until it comes naturally: "*I have no idea what you're talking about. Please explain it to me.*" Try it in the mirror or with your dog or cat.
- Any time your consent to a medical procedure is requested, inquire about the availability of alternative treatments, less invasive options or the potential health care outcome if you choose watchful waiting. If your consent is *not* requested, find out why.
- In case you are not quite ready to make a decision or proceed, don't. Authorizing a medical treatment is up to you, not the doctor, not the surgery scheduler and not the hospital social worker. Being health literate will give you the confidence to advocate for yourself or for someone else.
- Yes, you do have a permanent record and everything about your health care is in it or should be. Under HIPAA (the *Health Insurance Portability and Accountability Act*), you have the right to see your medical records, obtain a copy for a reasonable charge and request any necessary corrections be made.
- You're entitled to a copy of your medical records because you own the contents; the provider owns the media. You might be surprised to learn who owns the health care facility and who your provider works for. Ask if you want to know.

- For vulnerable populations, advocacy and direct care are already compromised due to dwindling resources at all levels. Do *not* depend on institutional oversight or regulatory agencies to keep vulnerable persons safe.
- Does your primary care provider or specialist make hospital rounds? If not, how is that handled if you're hospitalized? *Right now* find out how best to establish communication between hospital personnel and your usual providers in the event of hospitalization. Write it down where you or your proxy can find it when needed.
- For a hospitalized patient, double-check and address all the following: wrist band information; charted names of providers, health care proxies and emergency contacts; whether the patient can handle self-care issues, such as getting out of bed, ordering meals or calling for a nurse; and the accuracy and visibility of special orders or status records, e.g., allergies, do-not-resuscitate order, no visitors, food restrictions.
- When a new prescription is recommended, give it the same shared decision making scrutiny any medical treatment deserves. (See Chapter Fifteen for details.)
- If a second opinion is warranted, find out what medical records will be forwarded and then double-check all are ultimately received by the second provider. Inquire about the advisability of having medical tests readministered for the benefit of the second opinion doctor.
- Do not transition from one level of care to another, e.g., from the emergency department to a room or from the hospital to home or rehab, without having clear verbal and written communication about what was done and what needs to happen next. (See Chapter Sixteen for more about *care handoffs*.)
- If we learned nothing else from the pandemic, we know washing hands makes a difference. Patient safety may require courage. Those who enter your exam room or hospital room to treat you should wash up or glove up.
- It's customary to introduce ourselves when we meet someone for the first time. The same is true in health care, except how quickly the other person gets to know you can be a matter of life or death. Have an up-to-date medical profile in writing or on a smartphone app ready to share with a new provider or in an emergency.
- If more than one first-degree relative (parent, sibling or child) develops the same cancer, a family member contracts cancer at an early age, there's an increased risk due to one's ethnic background or an abnormal test result suggests the possibility of an inherited condition, each is the warning of a potential genetic link. Discuss how an aspect of one's medical history impacts preventive care, and make cautionary notes a permanent part of the medical record.[333]

- If you're not asked about an element of your medical or personal story you believe may be relevant, volunteer the information, e.g., a veteran subjected to possible service-related health risks or someone with a unique family history.
- Whenever you're unable to advocate for yourself, your appointed health care proxy is your voice and medical storyteller. Get the damned paperwork done.

When I need a break, I sometimes go to a Jim Gaffigan video until I'm ready to get back to work. Just as I was writing this chapter, I came across an interview with Jim and his wife Jeannie about the brain tumor she was successfully treated for in 2017. Jeannie learned about the "large mass" on her MRI and the doctor then said, "*I'm not a neurosurgeon, so here's some phone numbers. Tell them I referred you from this MRI. Go to the radiology center. Get your scan. And bring it to the appointment.*" I think you'd agree this health care professional may want to aim a bit higher when communicating life-altering and mind-numbing news. The Gaffigans were left in limbo.

Jim's advice for moving forward hit home as I wrote about self-advocacy: "*Make a plan. That's what you have to do. You have to make the best next decision you can make. And so that's what we did.*"[334] He is absolutely right. You must aim for the best next decision *you* can make under the circumstances, after gathering all the information and input it takes for *you* to be fully informed. And it is simply not possible to achieve that goal while remaining invisible.

Many forces are working to shift our roles from *patient to pawn.* We are complicit unless and until we claim our rights and responsibilities as masters of our health care fate. If you want to be seen—and heard—start by losing the cloak of invisibility.

CHAPTER THIRTEEN

Death: the ultimate adverse event

Increased complexity leads to increased risks. Health care is a prime example. If both patients and practitioners would come to recognize that most medical errors can be prevented by practicing the fundamentals of health literacy, it would be a powerful tool for conserving resources—and saving lives.

More than an occasional missing sponge

By now, you've gathered I believe in reliable sources. For instance, I would never use 37-year-old research to make the case for anything related to health care, certainly not lethal medical errors. Others don't agree, as evidenced by their unwavering reliance on *To Err Is Human: Building a Safer Health System,* a 1999 report on the prevalence of medical errors from the Institute of Medicine (IOM).[335] You may recall the IOM is the nonprofit established by Congress to conduct research and advise the federal government on health care matters. More specifics in a bit, but first, definitions:

- A *medical error* is an act of omission or commission in health care planning or execution that contributes or could contribute to an unintended outcome, whether or not a patient is harmed as a result.
- An *adverse event* is injury to a patient resulting from health care management, rather than the patient's underlying disease or medical condition, that results in prolonged or additional treatment, disability or death. Not all are medical errors.[336]
- *Patient safety* is having processes in place to prevent or reduce the frequency and impact of adverse events and unnecessary harm in the delivery of health care.

Until now, you may have thought medical errors happen only when a doctor leaves a sponge behind or operates on the wrong body part or the wrong body. Those particularly egregious and harmful medical errors are called *sentinel events* or *never events* because one can only hope they never occur, although they do, an estimated 4,000 times a year.[337] They are sprinkled among the most commonly occurring medical errors:

1. A mistake during a test, surgery or treatment.
2. The misdiagnosis of a medical issue.
3. The wrong test, surgery or treatment.
4. An error in ordering or dosing medication.
5. Wrong or unclear follow-up care instructions.
6. Being injured or getting an infection while being treated.[338]

So besides the never events, there are a myriad of often events. They are the medical errors that happen frequently and can be every bit as devastating.

First measure, then improve

The first step in striving for patient safety is realizing nearly every action or inaction in the course of your health care journey has the potential of triggering a medical error. An estimated 20 to 40 percent of Americans have experienced a medical error, either personally or secondhand alongside someone close.[339] Thankfully, not all medical errors result in the patient being harmed or the patient's treatment being negatively impacted. The medical errors that don't result in serious harm are known as *near misses*, *close calls* or *potential adverse events*.[340] Nevertheless, with more than 36 million hospital admissions each year, there's still a huge potential for a medical error to become an injurious event.[341] Studies have estimated 251,000 to 400,000 Americans lose their lives to medical errors each year.[342] If true, medical errors are our third leading cause of death, right behind heart disease and cancer.[343] That is problematic.

Okay, yes, it's also about the money. Globally, 15 percent of all hospital activity and expenditures are attributed to medical errors.[344] In the United States, annual costs from medical errors fall between $20 billion and $100 billion per year;[345] preventable harm from improper medications alone costs $21 billion to $40 billion each year.[346]

To put the categories of medical errors into practical terms, here's a sampling of research findings concerning types and frequency:

- Mistaken diagnoses occur in 5 to 10 percent of all medical conditions; AHRQ asserts one third of patients experience a diagnostic error first-hand and 80,000 persons die annually as a result; in vascular events, infections and cancers, it's 10 percent, suggesting they cause 40,000 to 80,000 deaths per year.[347]
- Second opinions result in either a completely different or a redefined diagnosis in the great majority of cases.[348]
- Patients omit doses, mix incompatible drugs or store meds incorrectly, reducing the effectiveness of medications or even causing an adverse drug event (ADE).[349]
- Auto-filled medications continue to be delivered to a patient, even though the drug has been discontinued by the prescribing physician.[350]
- Less than half of patients suffering a traumatic brain injury receive effective aftercare instructions or a follow up visit with a neurologist or any provider.[351]
- Patients experience a hospital-acquired infection (HAI) more than a million times every year. That's 650,000 hospitalized patients, one in every 25.[352]
- Direct patient care professionals comply with recommended hand hygiene standards less than half the time (a prepandemic study), despite the known benefits of hand-washing in preventing infection for the past nearly 200 years.[353]

- An estimated 2.5 million injuries result annually from hospital-acquired pressure ulcers (aka bedsores).[354]

When the IOM released its 312-page report *To Err Is Human* in 1999, it was monumental, judging from the publicity it received then and the respect it has since garnered.[355] It's intriguing that such a revered authority—cited more than any other source on the subject of medical errors—presented no data of its own and relied on three states' research to justify its nationwide inferences. Those studies were already seven to 15 years old in 1999.[356] Even allowing for the passage of time, the IOM's estimates of 44,000 to 98,000 annual deaths from in-hospital medical errors remain in stark contrast to recent independent research putting fatalities in the hundreds of thousands. Nevertheless, HHS continues to rely on those 1999 IOM statistics as its benchmark for strategic planning, public messaging, industry education and compliance concerning the issue of patient safety—well, at least until December 2020.

That's when, out of the blue, AHRQ began floating the notion that the number of deaths due to medical errors may actually be fewer than 4,000 a year.[357] Talk about confusing. AHRQ staff concurrently reports there are 80,000 deaths each year from misdiagnoses, just one type of medical error.[358] Tough to know what to make of that.

Here's the closest we have to data on deaths caused by some of the more common categories of medical errors. These statistics come from the HHS subagencies of AHRQ, CDC, CMS and NIH, as well as studies by independent researchers:

- Sepsis: 270,000 annual deaths.[359]
- Surgery site infections: 6,000 to 12,000 annual deaths.[360]
- Hospital-acquired pressure ulcers: 60,000 annual deaths.[361]
- Medication errors: 7,000 to 9,000 annual deaths.[362]
- Mistaken diagnoses: 80,000 to 99,000 annual deaths.[363]

Except for medication errors, these reflect fatalities only among hospitalized patients. We don't track medical error deaths in other settings, such as clinics, nursing homes and rehabilitation hospitals. Truth be told, we don't really track medical errors at all, only the occurrence of some patient injuries that may or may not result from medical errors. For instance, some might argue not all hospital-acquired conditions (HACs) are medical errors, e.g., sepsis, surgery site infections and pressure ulcers. However, according to the health care industry's own definitions, if an adverse event is preventable, it's a medical error. So how many of the deaths from HACs listed above were preventable? Impossible to say, again, because the industry doesn't track medical errors as a contributing cause of death, let alone the specific circumstances. Regardless, deaths attributable to causes that *are* tracked total considerably more than 4,000, or even 98,000—200,000 to 300,000 more by HHS's own reckoning. This gives you some idea of the magnitude of medical error fatalities, which is scary as hell. Experts can continue to argue the veracity of these conflicting estimates and no doubt will. Whether or not medical errors are the third leading cause of death in America, if you're a victim, it could be Number One for you. Let's see what we can figure out on our own about why these errors occur.

It's not too difficult to spot some reasons

To Err is Human was not only the premier attempt to quantify deaths from medical errors but also first to offer causes and solutions. Its general conclusion was that medical errors occur because *health care services is a complex and technological industry prone to accidents.*[364] Read: stuff happens. Viewing patient safety as largely a systems issue to be resolved with systems solutions leaves patients with no guidance in taking direct and practical steps to prevent harm. You know by now I don't agree we should let that stand in the way of being engaged and safe. Although the meager data we have on medical errors doesn't usually include the underlying cause, you and I can still recognize obvious triggers and be proactive in prevention. Let's look at just one.

The IOM definition of a diagnostic error includes the failure to fully explain the health care issue to the patient.[365] Sure enough, more than one third of the top 20 factors contributing to medical errors relate directly to failures in disclosure and consent, such as doctors not listening and patients not understanding.[366] This, even though we know disregarding these patient rights is a costly and ethically unacceptable lapse. While not all medical errors are preventable, those caused by failures to communicate are actionable opportunities for improvement, on both sides of the exam table.

We can also find contributing factors in health care's perfect storm. First, demographics, where aging and chronic conditions lead to more frequent use of health care resources, which increases the chance of errors. Similarly, the complexity and logistics of treatment options make patients more vulnerable to miscalculations and misjudgments. Second, resources. What portion of medical errors are caused by labor and financial shortages? Some measure of quality control must be sacrificed when those responsible for oversight are missing. Understaffing leads to overworking, which reduces time for shared decision making, and no reasonable person would argue a distracted or pressured health care professional is working to full and attentive capacity. Also, we don't have to guess whether providers' levels of stress and burnout impact their ability to facilitate communication and avoid errors—we're already seeing that. Then we come to the third element, patients and advocates failing to practice the health literate engagement needed for self-preservation. That's us, and it's where we can work to make the health care journey safer, in spite of overarching systemic influences that are certainly out of our control.

Yes, stuff happens in an undertaking as complex as health care largely dependent on human beings for management and delivery. Providers are often without the time, energy and interactive skills to fully implement quality control measures and to properly involve patients in shared decision making. Likewise, most health care consumers aren't trained to be engaged care management partners. It's just a fact: Responsibility for some portion of harmful adverse events—certainly medication errors come to mind—lies entirely at the feet of health care consumers. At the same time, our awareness and mindfulness can safeguard us against many mistakes. Because demographics and resources are not ours to manipulate does not preclude our ability to address manageable risks through health literate practices. We have to ask ourselves, *Are stakeholders, clinicians, policy makers and patients using all we know to advance the goal of patient safety?*

What is the prognosis for keeping patients safe?

The IOM's *To Err Is Human* proposed local, state and national agendas to promote patient safety, declaring in 1999, "*The status quo is not acceptable and cannot be tolerated any longer.*" Its vision for patient safety in the new millennium included 1) a federal clearinghouse for the development of patient safety leadership, research, tools, protocols and education; 2) nationwide mandatory and voluntary reporting of medical errors by health care providers; 3) raising standards and expectations through policy makers, stakeholders, oversight organizations and professional groups; and 4) fostering a culture of safety through the implementation of practices already proven in other industries.[367] More than twenty years later, how's it going?

First, the IOM report spawned the *Healthcare Research Quality Act* of 1999, which authorized the Agency for Healthcare Research and Quality (AHRQ) under HHS, where it continues to reside. It is "*the lead federal agency charged with improving the safety and quality of America's health care system.*"[368] With an annual budget of $338 million, AHRQ is slated to become part of the National Institutes of Health in 2021, which has its own budget of $41 billion.[369] Yes, this is the same AHRQ responsible for the compilation and projection of health care workforce data. (A corresponding agency, the National Center for Patient Safety at the Veterans Health Administration, was also formed in 1999 with an annual budget of $7.4 million.[370])

Second, as for establishing a federal mandate for reporting medical errors, there still isn't one. When that was proposed in 1999, 15 states already had their own laws addressing this issue, a number that grew to 28 in the seven years following the publication of *To Err is Human*—and then stopped.[371] CMS requires Medicare and Medicaid providers to report hospital-acquired conditions, just one category of adverse events. However, only 37 states have their own mandates echoing CMS requirements, and although individual states can choose to track data gathered under the federal program, most do not.[372] It hasn't been established whether there is any correlation between having available data on previous adverse events and a subsequent reduction in numbers. But we do know that if medical error reporting had been required back when first recommended by the IOM, we would now have more than two decades of hard data to use in implementing preventive measures, if so inclined.

As for the IOM's third objective, has a climate of patient safety been encouraged among industry stakeholders and professional groups? In 2015, 16 years after publishing *To Err Is Human*, the IOM issued a 444-page sequel entitled *Improving Diagnosis in Health Care*. It concluded that *misdiagnoses,* one narrow category of medical errors, had been "*largely unappreciated in efforts to improve the quality and safety of health care.*"[373] No kidding. Nevertheless, as we educate the internists of tomorrow, an average of only 6.4 hours is devoted to clinical reasoning, which is the art and science of diagnosing medical conditions. More than half of surveyed medical schools dedicate *no* teaching sessions to diagnostic reasoning.[374] It is assumed those skills will be acquired during the students' hospital residencies—as if willing mentors have the time.

That brings us to the IOM's final goal, which was to learn from other industries' established safety efforts, and aviation is one of the places it looked to study the concept of checklists. I'm not a health care professional, so like most consumers, I assume a lot about what's behind the curtain. I know I need written prompts to have a successful trip to the grocery store, so when I heard the World Health Organization had created a pioneering *Surgical Safety Checklist*, it made perfect sense. It takes about two minutes to complete and includes items such as the patient's identity at the start and a sponge count at the end. Then I learned Dr. Atul Gawande of *Being Mortal* fame had assisted in its development and I got to thinking, *Dr. Gawande's not an old guy, so he must have been a kid when he worked on this, right?* About then I discovered the surgery safety checklist was developed in 2008. It had taken nearly 250 years for stakeholders to acknowledge this gap in safety and attempt to plug it. Another thing we always thought was handled, but wasn't.

The great news is, this checklist has been shown to dramatically reduce postoperative deaths. However, as one medical expert observed, "*There is evidence to support that the positive effect of a surgical safety checklist relies on systematic implementation.*"[375] An obvious truth, it would seem: Checklists only work when actually used. They are now employed in almost 90 percent of surgeries in the United States each year, which is a lot, but that still leaves about 6.5 million times when the potential for a *never event* still exists.[376] Baffling.

In furtherance of patient safety, the Centers for Medicare and Medicaid Services began to identify categories of hospital-acquired conditions (HACs) in 2008. These adverse events include infections, leaving foreign objects behind in a surgery (where's a checklist when you need one?), air embolisms, post surgery blood clots and serious falls.[377] Medicare providers reporting a patient with a medical condition or injury acquired in the hospital find themselves with lowered reimbursement rates. Honestly though, there's not a great history of success using such disincentives. From 2010 to 2016, Medicare's financial penalties intended to reduce what are viewed as preventable hospital readmissions within 30 days resulted in an impressive one percent drop.[378]

Sepsis is a single type of infection among HAIs. It infects between 1.7 and 2.7 million persons annually, costs $41.4 billion in the care of Medicare patients alone and causes 270,000 deaths each year, according to HHS. In fact, one in three persons who dies in a hospital has sepsis at the time of death.[379] What percentage of sepsis cases are health care-acquired and preventable adverse events? Good questions. To boost preventive efforts, HHS formed the *Federal Steering Committee for the Prevention of Health Care-Associated Infections* (HAIs) in 2008 with the ambitious mission of overseeing 15 working groups from public and private sectors to identify new approaches to HAI prevention. It formulated a national action plan in 2013 and then, crickets. When asked to disclose the membership roster, activities and accomplishments of this advisory group since its 2008 inception, the supervising federal agency responded that the Steering Committee is meeting to review data and "*does not have anything additional to share publically* [sic] *on their activities at this time.*"[380] That's okay, we are already certain of two things: 1) the often-cited statistic of 99,000 deaths per year from HAIs is based on data from 2002 and 2) handwashing is the most effective way to prevent sepsis.[381]

If you sense not everything possible is being done to keep us from unintended and/or preventable harm while receiving medical care, you are spot on. Hospital-acquired pressure ulcers, aka bed sores, are another example of good research gone nowhere. Multiple government and private sources tell us 2.5 million patients suffer from these injuries each year and 60,000 do not survive (1989 data). To dispel any question about their preventability, a 2019-20 study implemented a concentrated effort to avoid pressure sores at three hospitals. It resulted in more than a 60 percent reduction in harm.[382] That was just three of America's 6,100 hospitals, but it was a start.

When we compare Americans' experiences with medical errors today, compared to 20 years earlier, we find:

- Sixteen percent *fewer* patients receive medical treatment as disclosed to them.
- Nineteen percent *fewer* get sufficient instructions for taking a medication.
- And this is the killer—literally—25 percent *fewer* receive an accurate diagnosis.[383]

In 2019, Gopal Khanna, the director of AHRQ, marked the 20th anniversary of *To Err is Human* by first praising his agency's impressive record, measured by $3.1 billion spent on 3,900 research grants cited in more than 27,000 articles. Khanna then acknowledged that a single category of medical errors, diagnostic mistakes, affects an estimated 12 million patients every year in America. While not all misdiagnoses result in patient injury, Khanna claims one third of those patients—four million individuals—*do* suffer serious harm from misdiagnoses. The estimated annual cost of that single category of medical errors: $100 billion.

And what are AHRQ's "*bold plans*" to address this crisis in mistaken diagnoses going forward? Khanna says, "*Our initial work should focus on the three largest areas of diagnostic errors: cancer, vascular conditions, and infections*."[384] "*Initial work*"? More than 22 years ago, *To Err Is Human* identified *mistaken diagnoses* as one of the most frequently occurring medical errors. Six years ago, AHRQ helped to fund the IOM's 2015 follow-up report, *Improving Diagnosis in Health Care,* which was devoted exclusively to the widespread dangers of diagnostic errors. Here we are, $3.1 billion and nearly four thousand research projects later and leadership at AHRQ is mulling over the "*initial work*" needed to stop these deadly medical missteps? No way.

We should not be surprised, since AHRQ recently reported less than half of its targeted patient safety measures showed improvement from 2000 to 2018. Less than half. True to form, their priorities are clear: If there's any hope of improving patient safety, we will need more studies. To that end, AHRQ has hired private health care-related entities under a contract with a potential value of $175 million to develop a "*call to action*" on—wait for it—how to help health care executives adopt a "*growth mindset*" to prioritize diagnosis safety. One of the first conclusions to be drawn by these industry leaders, who choose to rely on 2004 data, is that "*evidence suggests failures in diagnosis plague the general patient population*."[385] Can't argue with that. I have to say: From where you and I are sitting, the prognosis for patient safety isn't looking too good.

The music has stopped. Grab a chair.

What's the value in you and I knowing so much about adverse events and medical errors? First, these statistics reveal the magnitude of the risks to be avoided throughout our health care journeys. Second, they demonstrate how out of touch policy makers are with the true scope of the threat. Finally—and most importantly—the refusal of policy makers and stakeholders to properly acknowledge this lapse in patient safety reinforces our assumption that the duty of caution and prevention falls to us.

Cynical it may seem, but as patients and advocates, we should assume there is always the potential for unintended harm. Once you realize how many lives are impacted and taken every year by medical errors and adverse events, it may be difficult to imagine how the preventive actions of any one person can matter in the big scheme of things. I would argue that not only can individual patients, proxies and providers make a difference, by default they are first defenders in preserving patient safety.

Look again at the meaning of a medical error: *An act of omission or commission in health care planning or execution that contributes or could contribute to an unintended outcome, whether or not a patient is harmed as a result.* Some sources have adopted definitions that differ slightly, but no one assigns exclusive blame to the health care professionals. Think about it: Is it on the provider(s) or on the patient to oversee safe drug use when multiple physicians and multiple pharmacies are involved? If neither patient nor proxy discloses all symptoms and a diagnosis misses the mark, who committed the act of omission? Who threatens patient safety when a careless visitor fails to observe prudent hygiene practices in the clinic waiting room or hospital?

Policy makers and stakeholders prefer to lay blame at the feet of the nebulous health care *system* and its processes and conditions, rather than impugn the actions or inactions of individuals. Potential solutions are seen as opportunities to limit liability, rather than prevent adverse events. One saves money, the other, lives. This is how they're paid to think and I get that.[386] Meanwhile, the IOM made it clear patients are central to solving the problem of misdiagnoses, but gave us no marching orders. Consumers and individual practitioners don't have the bureaucratic or administrative authority to make systemic changes in the delivery of health care or reallocate resources for the sake of patient safety. We do, however, have this super power: For nearly every potential medical error, there is an available preemptive measure. Those on the front line of health care's safety battle—patients, proxies and providers—do have the ability to prevent many medical errors or at least to prevent harm.

Strategies for self-preservation / Medical errors

Many adverse events and medical errors can be routinely avoided by simply practicing the fundamentals of health literacy, including full disclosure and informed consent. The fully informed shared decision making that should occur prior to every health care treatment requires at least two participants. If either the provider or the patient is not fully engaged in that process, the chance of suffering a medical error rises dramatically.

There's a simple maxim that supersedes all preventive measures: *Trust but verify.* Sure, you've got a great doctor, but that's just one member of the team and one piece of the health literacy puzzle. The patient and the patient's network of human and informational resources are just as crucial. Maintaining vigilance all along your health care journey—as much as is humanly possible—is a large part of maintaining safety.

As we cover the top six medical errors and how best to not experience one, recall and ponder the three building blocks of health literacy that apply in all health care circumstances. Keep them in the back of your mind:

A. *Identify and access reliable health literacy resources.*

B. *Practice shared decision making.*

C. *Take documentation action steps.*

Here are preemptive measures that can prevent adverse events or keep them from becoming harmful if they do occur:

1. A mistake during a test, surgery or treatment

Be proactive by thoughtfully choosing the members of your health care team, appointing effective patient advocates in case of incapacity, being fully informed before granting consent and insisting on shared decision making.

- Fully understand the purpose, possible risks and potential outcomes of any proposed test or procedure.
- Inquire about the expertise and experience of the provider and facility, e.g., is an outpatient surgery center equipped to handle a medical emergency, such as a cardiac or respiratory crisis?
- Immediately question any unusual or unexpected symptoms or outcomes.

2. The misdiagnosis of a medical issue

Getting the right diagnosis starts with having a capable medical detective. Do your homework before choosing a primary care provider or specialist as diagnostician, and don't hesitate to make a change or seek supplemental counsel if needed.

- It is not insensitive or inappropriate to ask about a provider's prior experience in dealing with your medical condition. Be familiar with the credentials of any health care professional and seek the expertise of a board-certified physician until your diagnosis is certain and a treatment plan is in place.
- Second-rate communication is often the culprit, so provide a complete and up-to-date patient story, including medications, preexisting conditions and all symptoms.
- If you don't understand, keep asking until you do, and repeat back all important information (it's called the "teach-back" method of communication), including your understanding of what led to the diagnosis.
- Whether the news is good or not so good, get a copy of test results with the physician's notes as soon as possible and before a treatment plan is finalized; verify that all information on the report is accurate, e.g., date, identity, condition, etc.
- Getting a diagnosis and/or prognosis that's "good news" (read: not as devastating or invasive as what you were imagining) doesn't preclude getting a second opinion. Are test results reliable and definitive? A false *all clear* leaving you without the treatment you should have can be just as detrimental as bad news.

- Get a second opinion if the medical condition or treatment has life-threatening risks, if the diagnosis is uncertain, if the treatment is experimental, if required by insurance or if you get a funny feeling at the back of your head.
- A second opinion is an opportunity to bring additional expertise and/or treatment options to the table; not to question the competence of the initial provider but to have the best possible health outcomes.
- The decision to seek a second opinion should not depend on finances. If the cost of new tests or further consultation is an issue, explore options to do whatever is most likely to preserve patient safety and achieve the best health outcomes.

3. The wrong test, surgery or treatment

Remain engaged, keep any health care advocate up to date on the patient's medical history and treatment plan and question everything. Trust but verify.

- When you and your advocate fully understand your diagnosis and treatment plan, it increases the chances of detecting a medical error before it causes harm.
- In reviewing a consent form, concentrate on the parts that disclose known risks and identify the patient, the provider, the condition and the procedure.
- Volunteer the patient's name for verification prior to any test or procedure, confirm who ordered it and your understanding of the reason.
- If something doesn't sound or look right, speak up, share any unexpected symptoms or side effects and get resolution of all questions or concerns.
- In the case of multiple providers, request they establish and maintain a chain of communication to avoid treatment duplications or conflicts.
- Consider designating one provider as the care manager to oversee all tests and treatments and foster communication between multiple providers.

4. An error in ordering or dosing medication

Harm from medications is as likely to happen at the hands of the patient as the provider. Chapter Fifteen is devoted to the important topic of medications, but in the meantime, having a complete understanding of the what and why of all drugs you're taking is a good rule of thumb to protect you from many adverse drug events (ADEs).

5. Wrong or unclear follow-up care instructions

The most dangerous time in the life of a patient is the handoff between providers or different levels of care, such as going from the emergency department to a hospital room or from outpatient surgery to home or from your PCP to a specialist. Getting the handoff right is so crucial, it got its own chapter (Sixteen).

6. Being injured or getting an infection while being treated

Hospital-acquired conditions (HACs) are medical issues or injuries the patient did not have at admission and developed while hospitalized. They range the gambit from infections to falls. They can lead to additional or extended treatments, longer hospitalization, harmful complications and even death.

- Request that health care professionals double-check the patient's identity and all medical orders before administering any drug or test. Offer and verify multiple identifiers, such as the patient's name, address, social security, PCP, etc.
- For those with mobility issues or compromised physical or mental capacity, confirm help is available to avoid falls, wandering or anxiety from unfamiliar surroundings during hospitalization. Request a hospital sitter or arrange to stay with the patient.
- If you're unsure of your own stability, avoid falls by asking for help.
- Insist any attending health care workers—including doctors—either wash their hands or put on fresh gloves before attending the patient.
- Arrange for the patient's personal hygiene to be maintained, including keeping their hands clean, even if it requires the assistance of family members or the employment of additional caregiving workers.
- Know and watch for signs of infection associated with a catheter, central line, surgical site or wound.
- Make staff aware of any preexisting physical or mental health conditions that may exacerbate complications from the medical condition or treatment.
- Fully understand medical orders for physical activity and breathing therapy during and after hospitalization to avoid blood clots and pneumonia.
- For extended hospital or rehab stays, ask about the risk of pressure ulcers, practice preventive measures and be on the watch for associated symptoms.
- Hospital stays are for getting treated and getting well, not socializing, so reduce the risk of infections, unnecessary distractions and stress by limiting visitors.

". . . So, we no longer need to accept patient safety as what is estimated to be the third leading cause of death. We no longer have to accept that a third of patients will leave their health care interaction not knowing how to self-care, not feeling respected, not feeling they were listened to. And we'll stop squandering that third of every dollar on therapies that don't get patients well. That translates in the U.S. to over a trillion dollars, about $10,000 per household." (Peter Pronovost, Director, Johns Hopkins Hospital and Armstrong Institute for Patient Safety and Quality, June 2019)[387]

More than 20 years after medical errors were fully exposed as a systemic threat to achieving the best available health outcomes, the methods to prevent most adverse events remain obvious, actionable and cost effective. The failure of policy makers and stakeholders to fully protect the users of health care over the decades leaves only one remaining option for patients and advocates: Accept the responsibility to ask *Who? What? When? Where?* and *Why?* in every health care situation. It is but one more critical step in the process of choosing to not be a pawn.

CHAPTER FOURTEEN

Technology and the digital age

Along with life-saving and life-extending benefits, health care technology promised greater productivity, improved diagnostics and better care management. We got all that, but along with it came security breaches, provider burnout and higher risks for medical errors. Let's separate the hazards from the enhancements.

There was a time when getting a newspaper and mail twice a day and watching the 10:00 p.m. news was cutting edge media. If we still relied on only that, we would miss a lot. The 24/7 news cycle emits from an endless variety of online, satellite and app sources; the little speaker on the kitchen island responds to our every need (some we didn't even know we had); and a wristwatch nudges us to get in a few more steps. You cannot be the fully informed and engaged patient today's health care demands by using yesterday's logistics. This chapter introduces the language of health care technology and highlights the features that directly impact you as a patient or advocate.

We've come to use the term *technology* as shorthand for both *digital technology* and *information technology* (IT), which only adds to the general confusion. *Digital technology* is the use of programming code in computer-based products and solutions—it's on the developer side. For its end users, health care professionals and consumers, *information technology* uses those digital means to store, transmit and retrieve information. Health care technology embraces both, in the logistics and devices that record, track and treat medical issues, with the goal of improving quality of life for patients and providers. What follows here is an overview of technology's role in health care—today. I won't even pretend to vouch for tomorrow.

Alzheimer's Disease illustrates well the constant shifting of health care technology in diagnosis and treatment. The first symptoms of this dementia may be memory issues, confused thinking or difficulty in forming words. Choosing appropriate pharmacotherapy and making the right lifestyle decisions depend on having an accurate diagnosis. Twenty years ago, the only means of confirming suspicions was through an autopsy. Today, the starting point is still a clinical exam, including physical, mental and neurological evaluations, but there is so much more. Blood tests can pinpoint alternative causes for cognitive decline, i.e., a thyroid disorder or a vitamin deficiency; and a spinal tap or PET scan can detect levels of Alzheimer's amyloid markers. Brain imaging using an MRI or CT scan is available to eliminate another potential cause for symptoms, such as a stroke, brain trauma or tumor.[388] We now have specialized PET scans to distinguish between Alzheimer's and other dementias, and, most recently, there has been initial success with a blood test for Alzheimer's—a potential game changer in targeting an illness already ranked as America's sixth leading cause of death. As importantly, those tests may detect this disease even 20 years before symptoms first appear.[389] As for implementing the best treatment plan, telehealth solutions now include patient surveillance tools; exit and bed occupancy sensors; medication organizers; real-time online communication with caregivers; and nonpharmaceutical approaches to anxiety and confusion, such as music, light and aroma therapies.

Alzheimer's is just one example of how far we've come in using technology to achieve the best health outcomes and expand available options for reaching a patient's treatment and personal goals. It also illustrates the necessity for an effective advocate to be fully aware of available options. Technology is pervasive throughout our health care journeys, and knowledge is power. You're going to need all you can get.

Electronic health records

Every hospital records department and clinic reception area was once lined with walls of patient folders, color-coded and filled with sheaths of handwritten notes, x-ray film and paper EKG readouts. Today's *electronic health information* (EHI) includes *electronic health records* (EHRs), aka *electronic medical records* (EMRs). It all began as *clinical information systems*, crude databases when compared to the digitized systems now in use. The major push for EHR compliance began with the *Health Information Technology for Economic and Clinical Health Act* (HITECH), part of the *American Recovery and Reinvestment Act* of 2009. Converting to computerized records promised to cut red tape, reduce treatment/medication errors, enable data sharing and save billions of health care dollars. Health care provider EHR participation has since gone from 8 percent to 96 percent, a transition profoundly influenced by more than $38 billion in government incentives to hospitals, clinics and EHR software developers.[390] Motivated by this race to market, vendors paid too little attention to end users' real-life applications or the future interoperability of their systems. Except for the government's easily met "meaningful use criteria," there were no industry-wide format standards for EHRs. The result is a mishmash of EHR software products across the nation, most still in use today and largely not speaking to one another.[391] There's no nicer way to say it: EHRs have issues.

Lack of accuracy. Back in 2009, patient safety and efficiency were among the most enthusiastically promoted benefits of EHRs. Instead, research has found the inherent duplications, complexity and overwhelming volume of data make it nearly impossible to easily pinpoint information in real time, such as locating a patient's preexisting conditions, current medications or allergies in an EHR. Thirty-nine percent of tested systems fail to alert of a potential adverse drug event, discontinued prescriptions still appear to be active and 20 percent of EHRs contain errors.[392] An issue plaguing the entire system is *patient matching*, which means accurately accessing all medical data for a patient across provider or system portals. More about that in a bit.

EHRs are technology-dependent, but still rely on humans for their design and most of the data input and retrieval. By their very nature, EHRs are a contributing factor in provider burnout, as doctors spend nearly half their patient face time in data input, an emergency doctor can make an estimated 4,000 computer clicks during a single shift and pediatricians use 16 of each 21-minute appointment in EHR charting. When an EHR warns of a potential medical or medication hazard that doesn't really exist, providers begin to suffer from *alert fatigue* and stop paying attention. That creates a whole other source of risk when legitimate threats do occur. The patient safety element of EHRs is largely unregulated, so the frequency of medical errors is difficult to measure, except to conclude, "*Overall, substantial safety risk persists in current hospital EHR systems.*"[393]

Lack of interoperability. As each software developer generates a new EHR product, it is certified by the federal government for capability, functionality and security—but there is no current standard for *interoperability*. Simply put, the nearly 900 EHR systems being used by all manner of health care-related organizations don't work well with others. In fact, less than a third of hospitals can retrieve and integrate electronic patient information from outside providers—which is amazing, considering just two EHR vendors, Epic and Cerner, serve more than half of all hospitals in the United States.[394] When mergers and acquisitions occur, they bring additional layers of EHR systems under one organizational roof. This troubling lack of provider-to-provider communication doesn't even take into account facilities' internal conflicts, where the laboratory, medical records, patient portal, fundraising and billing departments may each have a stand-alone database and records—as can be said for every outside vendor. The IT equivalent of duct tape isn't working.

In existence since 1987, Health Level Seven International (HL7) is a private nonprofit that sets standards for the sharing, integration and retrieval of health data and patient records in the United States. It began addressing inter-provider digital communication issues in 2014.[395] Without getting too far into the weeds, in conjunction with CMS and HHS, HL7 has just launched massive changes to the federal government's standards for medical record access (131 pages of them). A series of steps moving toward full transferability and interoperability just began.[396]

First, *information blocking* rules go into effect, which prohibit practices standing in the way of exchanging, accessing or using electronic health information. That started April 5, 2021 and is intended to provide patients full access to their medical records, including providers' notes. It's already keeping clinic staffs busy responding to calls from patients seeking clarification and assurances concerning the puzzling test results and terminology they can now see in their EHRs. Insurers are required to enable open data exchanges by 2022; and, in theory, there will be full and transparent communication between all EHR systems by 2023.[397] Uh, maybe. In October of 2019, a survey showed less than one in five health care executives and slightly more than one fourth of insurers were *very familiar* with these quickly approaching deadlines, first proposed in the 2016 *21st Century Cures Act*.[398] Won't the rest be surprised? It is difficult—if not impossible—to see how the health care industry will overcome all obstacles to interoperability by the end of 2023, considering more than 70 percent of hospitals are currently unable to integrate data from other providers. The Department of Veterans Affairs was one of the first health care systems to implement EHRs, back in the 1970s. The VA has just begun the process of revamping its entire system at a cost of $16 billion, so far. Full implementation is scheduled to take *ten years*.[399]

The concern for you and me is whether there will be timely and accurate access to information needed by our providers and us to make smart and safe health care decisions. If you see four specialists, there's at least four points of entry for EHRs and at least four opportunities for errors and omissions. Yikes.

Lack of security. How does a simple car break-in cost one health care provider more than $1 million in fines? HIPAA (the *Health Insurance Portability and Accountability Act*) is more than just a name to drop when you want a copy of your medical records. Since 2009, HIPAA-covered entities are supposed to keep all patient health information from being accessed, used or read by unauthorized parties. That's why the volume is turned up on the waiting room television, to mask the receptionist's HIPAA-protected phone conversations; and that's why the theft of an unencrypted laptop from the car of a provider employee was newsworthy.[400] HHS—and the public—came to know about that break-in because HIPAA-covered entities are required by law to notify the government, affected patients and the media whenever a breach of protected health information includes the records of 500 or more individuals.[401] How often are such breaches reported and made public?

Let's just say the past few years have been good for hackers and bad for health care data security. There were 642 reported breaches of 500+ individuals' records in 2020, exposing more than 29 million patients' confidential medical info. The 2020 number of reported breaches is 25 percent larger than in 2019, which had 37 percent more than 2018. As for the actual volume of patients whose records were exposed, the 41.3 million individuals affected in 2019 was three times as many as in 2018 and more than the combined total of the previous three years. Big health care means big breaches, and more than half of the records exposed in 2019 were stored at just two entities.[402]

Since this reporting requirement was added to HIPAA in 2009, more than 266 million EHRs have been lost, exposed or disclosed in violation of HIPAA.[403] We can only hope we never again approach 2015's record setting 114.3 million compromised records, which included the granddaddy of all breaches—to date. *Phishing* is using a fake email to gain access through someone with legitimate IT credentials. An employee of health insurer Anthem's subsidiary innocently opened such an email and exposed the private medical information of 78.8 million customers.[404] Ouch.

Although health care provider organizations accounted for more than three fourths of 2020's breaches,[405] it isn't just medical professionals and payers who potentially jeopardize the safety of your confidential medical information. Similar risks originate from linked business peers, such as legal and accounting firms. A failure at a collection agency, AMCA, implicated 24 other associated entities, exposing more than 26 million medical patients' records. A provider of vision benefits to other insurers caused a data breach of 485,000 insureds' records in 2020, potentially including social security numbers, birth and marriage certificates and medical details.[406] Breaches even involve the suppliers of cybersecurity. While providing data storage for health care and fundraising entities, cloud service vendor Blackbaud allowed hackers access for nearly four months before discovery. The initial reported breach of less than one million client records has since been adjusted to more than ten million, including individuals' bank account information, user names, passwords and Social Security numbers.[407] More than enough data to build an incalculable treasure of assets and new identities. And breaches make individuals susceptible to *spear phishing*, which is using follow-up fraudulent emails to target specific individuals from the pool of stolen data, based on those patients' unique characteristics and medical information.

What allows these lapses in security to occur in the first place? It can be as simple as an employee using an unauthorized app on a company device, weak passwords, bad storage/improper disposal of records or a provider's failure to log out after accessing a network. On a larger scale, it might be using inadequate tools for scanning, encryption and filtering of emails; or having an inefficient backup system—or none at all. Of course, some security gaffes are less sophisticated, say, like the organization that off-loaded paper medical records to a dump site—a real dump, not a virtual dump—exposing the privacy of more than 550,000 patients.[408] In reviewing what we know about the biggest fails of 2020, the overwhelming majority, two thirds, came from outside sources hacking into the software. They include phishing and *ransomware*, in which malicious software blocks the provider's access to their own data until real money—or cyber cash—is paid to the hacker (think Colonial Pipeline and meat processor JBS). In 2019, ransomware attacks increased in frequency by 350 percent over 2018's volume,[409] and now account for almost half of all security breaches.[410] Here's a concept I just learned of and I'm sharing because it's so fascinating to me, a non-techie: A *zero-day vulnerability* is a software security flaw the developer knows about but hasn't yet figured out how to fix. The term comes from the fact that without a software patch at the ready, there are *zero days* to stop damage once hackers also discover it. Sometimes the bad guys just know stuff the good guys don't.

And private entities aren't the only ones exposing records by leaving an EHR system's back door open. The Marketplace software used by the federal Centers for Medicare and Medicaid Services was hacked in October of 2018, granting access to the personal information of 75,000 individuals. The same HHS subagency had to take its *Blue Button 2.0* health care app offline soon after launch when outsiders were kind enough to let the agency know it had a major leak. Previously undiscovered because CMS failed to conduct a prerelease test run, *Blue Button 2.0* is a potential portal to the records of 53 million Medicare beneficiaries. Not quite 78.8 million, but still.[411]

Lack of respect. Electronic health records are a virtual gold mine. With birthdates, credit cards, Social Security numbers, email addresses, phone numbers, emergency contacts, health insurance info and even photo IDs and scanned legal documents, hackers count each medical record a valuable commodity. A stolen identity can resell for over $1,000 a pop or be used for subsequent phone or online money scams. That's why our health care data is vended in bulk on the black market/dark web, e.g., one source was openly offering 397 patient records from a Georgia hospital.[412] And there's plenty of pitching going on in plain sight as well. A study of 821 medication phone apps found nearly eight in ten share their user data, i.e., they are dealing in your health care information.[413] I recently received an email telling me my emergency medical information app had been sold to a pharmacy chain. Although I was "invited" to transfer my data to the new owner, that had already been done, without any express consent from me. I closed the account, but I have no doubt my data lives on, in the hands of who-knows-who. Let's get real, the pharmacy was buying personal medical data, not a smartphone app nearly anyone can create using a YouTube instructional video.

Will the next keeper of your personal information and medical records be as security conscious as you would like? In August of 2019, giant EHR developer Epic announced the launch of Cosmos, a massive data compilation project for the ultimate purpose of medical research. Epic had an initial goal of gathering 20 million patient files from among the EHRs stored with its institutional clients. Just one year later, Epic had already deposited three times that number of records into the Cosmos data bank.[414] Although these EHRs are now described as *anonymous*, the fact that two thirds of Americans have data with Epic certainly gives a person pause. Before you even ask, yes, somewhere in the "Privacy Policy" you electronically signed—but didn't read—you gave your consent. It has even been suggested patients may want to consider whether they deserve royalties from those who so freely loan, sell and use their medical information, sort of like iTunes.[415] Yeah, that's probably not gonna happen. What's a patient to do?

If you can't say something nice . . .

. . . then you may be talking about EHRs. Electronic health records are a source of annoyance, frustration and downright danger for those compelled to interact with and depend on them—that's providers and patients. To remain safe while achieving the best health outcomes, we need to first acknowledge their shortcomings. It's noteworthy that four of 2020's top ten health technology hazards were EHR-related: alarm overload, cybersecurity risks in home health care, missing device implant data and medication dosing mistakes.[416] Really, except for those who get paid to design and redesign them, it's tough to find anyone who speaks well of EHR systems. It probably won't be you or me because we've experienced the frustration of repeatedly correcting misinformation. And certainly not once we figured out they contribute to doctor and nurse burnout by sucking up one fourth to one half of the energy that could be otherwise dedicated to patient interaction. Hey, that's our valuable provider face time they're messing with. Bad attitudes about EHRs clearly abound and when the people directly involved with our health care are unhappy, everyone suffers.

As a single example, providers are often forced to access multiple infosystems that don't cross communicate, each requiring logging in and logging out. These obstacles exist largely because EHRs were designed as digital versions of paper records, rather than data solutions intended to support and enhance patient-centered care.

- More than half of surveyed doctors believe EHRs have a negative impact on the doctor-patient relationship, as well as on providers' productivity.
- Seven out of ten providers think EHRs contribute to burnout.
- Those using EHRs have less job satisfaction and experience higher stress.
- EHRs are considered the least satisfying part of practicing medicine.
- Sixty percent of physicians think EHRs need a complete overhaul.[417]

The process that consumes half their professional life, the recordkeeping system doctors and nurses rely on to make life-and-death diagnoses and to guide treatment plans, is not even worth salvaging? Disturbing, but not surprising. Provider usability has been a low priority in the development of EHRs since their inception.[418] As consumers, we have little alternative but to accept that our medical record is adrift on a sea of bytes and to arm ourselves against the inherent risks.

Are you sure you're who you think you are?

Patient identifiers are morsels of information used to set one patient record apart from another. Traditionally, they've been chosen from among the individual's name, medical record number, date of birth, phone number, Social Security number, address and photo. *Smith, Johnson, Williams, Brown and Jones* are the most common surnames in the United States. If your name is John Smith, there's a good chance there's another John Smith in the patient database born on the same day as you. One hospital system in Harris County, Texas tested this theory. Of 3.4 million patients, two or more shared the same first and last names nearly 250,000 times; more than 69,000 also had the same date of birth.[419] What are the odds of a medical record mix-up? *Houston, we have a problem.*

Patient matching—or the lack of it—is where it all begins. It's the ability to accurately link a patient's records within and across data systems. In other words, it makes sure complete and accurate EHRs are "seen" and accessed during my care. If I'm "Jo" in one place and "Johannah" in the next, maybe no go. Or if the record of a previous medical procedure shows a former street address. For as long as we've had electronic health records, deficiencies in patient matching have been included in the Top Ten of patient safety concerns. When data is shared between related health care entities—even those using the same EHR developer—the match rate has been found to be as low as 50 percent. Failure to match means duplicate records occur for nearly one in every ten patients in the same health care facility, 86 percent of surveyed health care professionals say they personally know of a medical error resulting from patient misidentification, more than one third of identifier errors occur during diagnosis and one fifth of patient matching missteps involve patient treatments.[420] Life-and-death stuff.

Misidentification can originate from simple typos; changes in data after a move, marriage or divorce; and conflicting methods of entering names and addresses across EHR systems. The most common mismatches are attached to middle names, Social Security numbers and misspellings.[421] The system's inability to find the correct record can result in accessing the wrong patient's EHR, then updating it with someone else's medical history. Thanks to the interoperability that does exist, an error is then cyber dispersed throughout a patient's medical universe in a nano second. A few months ago, my phone number was apparently typed into the medical record of a stranger locally hospitalized, which may have happened at check-in, where 63 percent of misidentifications begin.[422] I started getting calls and texts throughout the day from pharmacists, rehab therapists, specialists and medical supply stores. I couldn't get the error corrected, so future data searches using my phone number won't produce her EHR. A friend received test results of a very delicate and confidential nature for another person who happens to share the same first and last name—nothing else. And now the other person's record shows she received a copy of those results, which she did not.

Failures in patient matching and misidentification are caused by time pressures, insufficient training, excessive duplications and plain old human screwups. Motivated by these obvious shortcomings in electronic health data management, many have long argued for a *unique patient identifier* (UPI), such as an iris scan, thumbprint reader, palm scan or smart card. The hope is that when cross-checked with other identifiers, these would be as fool-proof as is humanly possible. HHS recognizes that "*The need for a unique patient identifier is urgent and essential.*" Who can argue with that? Indeed, as when a patient is denied life-saving CPR, although it's the guy in the next bed who really has the do-not-resuscitate order; the incorrect ED patient goes into surgery, while the unattended person dies; or the lady on the wrong gurney gets medicated. Since EHRs are about to be completely revamped to meet government interoperability regulations, it seems like an apt time to also tackle the patient identifier issue once and for all. Really, it's hard to see why anyone would consider doing the former without the latter, because that would make absolutely no sense. And yet . . .

Although HIPAA is best known for protecting patient privacy, the Act also includes health insurance portability for persons between jobs and rules about how health care data is coded and transferred among organizations and payers. The HHS warning I just mentioned about the "*urgent and essential*" need for a unique patient identifier standard? That alarm was sounded over 24 years ago, in *1997*, on the heels of the then-new HIPAA regulations. The regs mandated HHS to adopt a "*unique health identifier for each individual, employer, health plan and health care provider for use in the health care system,*" in anticipation of technology's mushrooming role in health care delivery and data management.[423] In 1997, it seemed prudent to adopt standards for a patient identification system ensuring *your* medical records are relied upon when caring for *you*. It seemed prudent because it was prudent. This is where it gets really weird.

Mandated under HIPAA, yes, but a mandate is only as viable as the funds committed for its implementation, as we've witnessed before. For more than 24 years, Congress has barred HHS from spending any federal money to promulgate or adopt a national standard for unique patient identifiers.[424] Another duh moment in legislative history. Understand, nothing has prevented private health care stakeholders from adopting patient identifiers they believe promote accurate patient matching. Some have done so; a great example is the Harris County, Texas system now using palm prints.

In 2017, health care-related organizations persuaded Congress to allow HHS to at least offer technical assistance to the private sector in coordinating a national strategy for patient identification standards. HHS saw a checkered flag and began spending millions on unique patient identifier—wait for it—*research*. Rest assured the Office of the National Coordinator for Health Information Technology (ONC) overseeing this system-wide concern is fully engaged in studying the issue. They even held a public contest in 2017 to get some good ideas for patient matching algorithms.[425]

In the meantime, the 1997 funding ban remains in place, originally premised on concerns for patient privacy. I'm just going to say that this justification concerning UPIs is overshadowed by the exposure of 266 million medical records through EHR security breaches over the past decade. Consider this: Just about the time the new interoperability rules for EHRs are fully implemented, we'll wish we had effective patient identifiers in place. Otherwise, how will all those EHR systems finally communicating with each other know for certain who they're talking about? Like I said, electronic health records are good for the folks who design and redesign them.

Strategies for self-preservation / Electronic health records

How stealthily over time the security of our medical records has been eroded. Although we had virtually no say in the design of the system, we find ourselves suffering from the failure of others to ensure accuracy and privacy. Because our health care is now so dependent on electronic health information, some level of risk is unavoidable. For instance, one in five security breaches is due to an employee error, but you and I don't control whether a provider's IT department is suitably staffed or supervised. If we did, we might first prohibit the opening of any email from a stranger, even if it holds the promise of a baby goat video (super cute).[426] As consumers, we can learn to be mindful of what's happening on *our* side of the curtain, and we must. Here are action steps to maintain watchfulness concerning EHRs:

- Find out how your provider(s) are implementing the new federal regulations relating to *information blocking* and seek their guidance on accessing physicians' notes and test results now available to you as a patient. Most importantly, learn how best to accurately interpret and respond to what you find in your EHR.
- Check for inaccuracies by regularly reviewing EHR highlights (e.g., chronic conditions, allergies, medications and preventive test results), at least once a year. Verify that corrections are made in the systems of all providers, associated or not.
- Do not assume your EHR will be accessed during an emergency, even at a facility where you've been treated before. You and/or your advocate should always have your medical history available to refer to and offer to providers.
- Review critical information whenever you meet a provider for the first time or are in an acute or emergency situation. *Never* assume an attending health care professional has up-to-date, accurate or complete medical information about you.
- If other potential targets of secondary hacking, such as credit cards and bank accounts, show unauthorized activity, it may indicate a breach of your EHR.
- If you need some or all of your medical records transferred for any reason, begin by asking what the process is to obtain your file and then verify the same at the receiving end. If electronic transfer is possible, it could happen digitally or you might need to hand carry a CD or flash drive.

- It's bizarre in light of all this tech talk, but you may find that a paper copy or fax of your records is the only way to move them from one provider to another.
- Try to obtain a written list of the exact tests, records, films, etc. being transmitted to the receiving specialist or provider.
- Once records have been transferred from one provider to another, verify their arrival and take inventory to make sure everything got there.
- Be prudent and request a copy of any transferred records for yourself; store the CD, flash drive or paper file in a safe place for future reference. Some patient portals allow you to download or print information, which is helpful, but there is no guarantee it's the same EHRs being accessed by your clinicians.
- There may be reasonable charges for transferring medical records on your behalf and there will definitely be delays, so be proactive by anticipating. Take a deep breath.

Let's focus on the most common patient matching issues and adopt provider-patient practices that minimize the chance of error or harm.

- *Incorrect patient identification upon admission.* The patient or advocate should volunteer multiple patient identifiers, such as name *and* address *and* date of birth; verify the medical reason for any admission, treatment, medication or test; check and double-check wristbands and test result labels for accuracy.
- *Time constraints during treatment.* Insist providers allow you the opportunity to confirm key information in your medical record, such as existing medications, allergies, medical devices, chronic conditions, recent procedures and the reason for the current visit, before proceeding.
- *Employees not aware or not properly trained.* Be patient, allow staff the time needed to confirm medical data and properly assess the situation before they act, and confirm any "next steps" before parting company.
- *Mistakes made while inputting data.* Verify, verify, verify by repeating back to staff any patient identifiers or medical orders; as needed, ask a second employee to review your medical record to confirm any corrections were made; ask to see any test order and review it with testing personnel before they begin.
- *Inadequate safety procedures.* Just as it is acceptable to ask someone to wash their hands before an examination or treatment, it is not out of line to double-check the accuracy of your medical records and verify patient matching. Ignore anyone who claims otherwise.[427]

If you view the top ten root causes of patient misidentification, almost all result from obvious and preventable human actions or inactions. There are specific measures available to stop or correct a misidentification before it becomes a medical error—and then an adverse event. Three suggestions for *health care personnel*:

- Triple verify patient identity prior to any procedure or medication.
- Proof chart notes before hitting the Enter key.
- Do not depend solely on information from patients with impaired cognition.

It's easy to see how reliance on technology and its promises of increased productivity have bred a false sense of security. As we begin to recognize known risks, we must acknowledge that not all errors are preventable at the point of direct patient care. No palm print will protect you from the wrong test being scanned into a medical record, as we learned from the patient who received someone else's cancer diagnosis, A system failure is preventable only through remedial measures on the system level. Still, as patients, advocates and providers, we can do what we can do. Yes, it takes extra effort to double-check and review patient medical records with professionals upon admission, before a procedure or at discharge. What value can be placed on the investment of time required to avoid having the wrong test, getting another person's medication or missing an important follow-up appointment?

Telehealth

Electronic medical records are just one element of health care technology, on the data management side. Technology has assumed an equally important role in patient care. There is often confusion between the terms *telehealth* and *telemedicine*, even among health care experts. To clarify:

Telehealth (also known as *telemonitoring* or *telemetry*) encompasses all information technology and telecommunications used to provide patient monitoring and direct care from afar, as well as long-distance data transfer and provider education. It affords access for information gathering, health assessment, diagnosis, intervention, consultation and supervision, from down the hall or across the globe.

Telemedicine is limited to the telehealth subcategory of remote clinical services, which is the delivery of direct patient care over a distance using technology. It's when a provider telecommunicates directly with a patient, and it involves a live health care professional present on one or both ends of the connection. So, while all telemedicine is telehealth, not all telehealth is telemedicine.[428]

The *Internet of Things* (IoT). I know you're thinking, "*That's not a thing*," but it truly is and I'm not the one who thought it up. It's a technology system in which data is transferred without the intervention of humans, and it has arrived, as measured by the presence of more objects than persons now hooked up to the Internet. Think driverless tractors, smart home security systems and wearable health monitors, which brings us to the *Internet of Medical Things* (IoMT).[429] You may be amazed at how technology is already being used to deliver health care in America's clinics, homes, care facilities and hospitals, which is just one element of telehealth. On this list, you might discover ways to achieve better health outcomes for yourself:

- Two parties, which could be any combination of patient, primary care provider, specialist, pharmacist, therapist or pathologist, consult by video, email or telephone.
- A digital record of a patient's clinical exam is forwarded to a remote provider using *asynchronous store-and-forward data transmission* of patient tests, records, photographs and video to be stored on the receiving end and reviewed in the future.
- A clinician uses voice recognition software to chart a medical record during examinations and consultations, freeing him from manual data input and allowing more time to focus on the patient and direct care.[430] We like the sound of that.
- Patients are monitored with *clinical-grade wearables,* which include pacemakers, implantable cardioverter defibrillators (ICDs) and vest ICDs; Blue Tooth-enabled smart inhalers use reminders and alerts to track medication dosage and usage; wristband apps upload medical data directly to an EHR vendor; a wearable device tracks blood pressure; and diabetic patients use insulin monitors and pumps to stabilize blood sugar levels.[431]
- *Remote patient monitoring* (RPM) offers tools to manage a chronic illness or post-discharge care, continuously or intermittently. *Medical telemetry* checks vitals and cardiac activity, tracks insulin levels, takes blood pressure readings and even issues medication and appointment reminders.
- *Consumer-grade wearables,* such as smart watches and smartphone apps, track activities, measure quality of sleep and monitor the rate and regularity of heart beats.
- A clinician delivers care off-site for chronic care management, transitional care or a house call using specialized tool kits that include portable technology to measure oxygen levels, weight, blood pressure and even conduct simple lab tests.[432]
- A tablet computer *avatar* transmits visual home health care oversight, while a remote human monitor interacts conversationally with the patient and can react in real time to any concerning observations.[433]
- Symptom-checking websites allow a patient to conduct a preliminary assessment of a medical condition and apply simple home remedies.[434]
- Online and phone app *patient portals* put patient and provider in direct communication as well as allow patients to monitor test results, track appointments, read providers' clinic notes and renew prescriptions. Although only half of patients say online access has been offered, once made available to them, more than half use the resource to access medical records.[435] The new HIPAA regs concerning patient access to EHRs will no doubt spawn more research.

- Telehealth/telemedicine systems used by EMTs transmit vital signs to the hospital from on-scene, evaluate stroke victims and can even translate a patient's native language while in route to the ED. This allows early intervention in the ambulance and optimal preparation at the trauma treatment site.
- More than 300,000 *mHealth* smartphone and tablet apps available for consumer use check symptoms, set pill reminders, record notes for the next doctor appointment and store vital health information for access in an emergency.
- On-demand videos educate patients on aftercare, medications, therapies and chronic illness management and can be viewed by the patient from home on a laptop computer, tablet or smartphone.
- For those homebound or with limited mobility, *personal emergency response systems* alert a central monitoring service in an emergency, including *smart belts* that detect falls in a hospital or home setting.
- A hospital uses IoMT smart devices to manage inventory, keep track of valuable equipment, regulate patient safety, control room temperature/humidity settings and even monitor how often employees wash their hands.
- Webinars and podcasts provide professional continuing education on new devices, medical procedures, software and research findings.[436]

Pretty cool, eh? In the time it's taken me to write this book, innumerable new technologies have been added to the menu. Keep in mind that what must remain unchanged are the basics of being informed, autonomous and safe.

Strategies for self-preservation / Telehealth

Anytime you have a health issue, it's in your best interests to learn about the latest available treatment and caregiving solutions. The list of available telehealth innovations demonstrates health care's rapid changes and the importance of engaged advocacy if you or a loved one are dealing with an acute or chronic medical condition. With twice as many American adults accessing the Internet as twenty years ago,[437] you may be researching a telehealth solution one day soon. Consider what systems or devices might make your best health outcomes more achievable, less stressful or safer. Exploring available technology is also a cue to seek expertise from your provider, working as a team in achieving both treatment and personal goals.

The importance of being your own best advocate must never wane. Technology presents unique challenges to patient safety. The changing face of telehealth may save provider time, but is there a cost? Here's a simple example: Your doctor decides to ditch his laptop and use voice recognition software for charting, with a microphone stashed somewhere in the exam room. Will it be time efficient for the provider and ultimately focus more attention on the patient? Probably, but who proofs the dictation to make sure *toes* isn't transcribed as *nose*? Is patient privacy sacrificed when those outside your doctor's clinic have access to verbatim conversations—legitimately or otherwise? How and how soon will that transcript be accessible in your EHR? If you want to keep part or all of a conversation off-record, thinking about the possibility ahead of time will strengthen your confidence to make the request. You *can* just say "no."

In all events, be a judicious consumer. Like in case you're tempted by the website where you pay to have *medical detectives* guess at a diagnosis for symptoms stumping your doctor. You can even sign up to be a sleuth yourself—it requires absolutely no health care expertise, just a giving heart and a deep desire to win a prize for the best guess. No, I am not kidding. Certainly, do not overlook the ubiquitous *smart assistants* or *chatbots*, like Siri, Alexa, Cortana and Google Assistant, available for a quick look-see. Nearly half of all Americans have used a digital assistant of some kind for advice about a health care issue. If you decide to go that route, you may want a second opinion. Studies have shown while most get it right some of the time, only some get it right most of the time and there are even instances when their counsel—and in no way is this meant to diminish their good intentions—can kill you.[438] Don't overlook the cyber chat rooms where people (in jammies) with the same illness as yours (or just too much time on their hands) will commiserate and counsel you for a fee. Not to worry about the website developers, they also get paid by those who buy your medical records from them.

Health care kiosks are another way of delivering remote health care services, both with and without human interaction. It may mean a computer tablet for patient check-in at the doctor's office, a video pod allowing patients to access EHRs or a station to verify temperatures prior to clinic admission during a pandemic. Kiosk solutions free up human resources for other duties and can include internet connections that measure vitals and manage medications. Maybe you've even used a blood pressure kiosk at your pharmacy. Self-serve kiosks in emergency departments shorten wait times and make more efficient use of staff for triage and treatment by linking the patient's check-in data with existing EHRs. But even sophisticated health care kiosks cannot fully replace human beings. They'll never know you as well as a trusted family member or best friend, or any human being using all five senses.

Telemedicine

You hear a soft buzzing, open your eyes and find a descendant of the Jetsons' Rosie at your hospital bedside. It's a two-wheeled video robot equipped for direct patient care.[439] Sometimes referred to as *remote clinical services, virtual care* or *telematics*, *telemedicine* is the clinical component of telehealth. A patient remains at a *spoke site* and receives a remote examination and care instructions from a human provider at the *hub site*. Communication may be through a smartphone, audio/video computer setup, A/V robot or specialized kiosk. Telemedicine can also be as simple as a phone interview. In this example of a bedside video robot, the spoke site is the patient's hospital room, while the hub site may be the nurses' station on that floor or in another state. Telemedicine can also mean a patient with a primary care provider who is consulting with a specialist via two-way video or telephone.

By the way, *virtual* is another term to be wary of in telehealth. Originally it meant the visual essence of something, but not the real thing. For instance, viewing the surface of the Moon through virtual reality goggles, as opposed to witnessing live coverage on July 20, 1969. The meaning is no longer so literal. Nowadays, although you refer to your video game buddy as your virtual friend, you know there really is a human being out there somewhere playing against you, even if you've never met for lattes. In health care, *virtual* generally means you're communicating with a real live person, even if you're seeing a computer-generated image on a video monitor, an *avatar*. My point is, make sure you're receiving patient care in real time. Verify there's a live doctor or nurse down the hallway or highway, not just the digital essence of a doctor, like Siri or Alexa.

Telemedicine may be newish to you and me, but it's been around since the 1960s when NASA developed it to monitor astronauts.[440] Fast forward to today. In a strange paradox, Medicare has reimbursed for telemedicine only in remote areas and then only if the patient travelled to a medical facility for the virtual appointment and the provider was willing to get paid less than for in-person consultations. Those most likely to benefit from this technology, elderly or mobility-challenged patients, were required to find transportation to the local hospital or clinic to see the remote doctor on a screen. Not surprising, rural and small-town providers who could put well-executed telemedicine to use are in health care facilities lacking the necessary training, transportation, funds, accessible EHRs and broadband services to embrace the technology. A classic Catch-22. The same is true for urban area community health centers serving lower income patients, where individual states determine the scope of Medicaid coverage. Under these restrictive guidelines, providers who desperately needed to supplement available staff with telemedicine failed to qualify for reimbursement.[441] Although a large majority of providers agree telemedicine is good for improved access and quality of care, only a very small proportion of clinics and patients had adopted its use over the decades. And then . . .

In March of 2020, everything changed, at least for a while. Prepandemic, there was a nationwide patchwork quilt of payer and public regulations for providing telehealth. Medicaid and private insurers varied widely on which telehealth services and devices were covered (i.e., live video, email, fax, telephone, store-and-forward EHRs and remote patient monitoring devices) and at what reimbursement rate. Furthermore, receiving health care remotely across state lines raised the question of medical licensure.[442] Along came COVID-19. Policy makers and stakeholders confronted with inescapable patient and provider safety issues were forced to find work-arounds to address staff and equipment shortages, not to mention the threat of contagion. (Coincidentally, when the pandemic struck, Medicare was already relaxing its reimbursement rules for remote patient monitoring, based on studies showing its value in improving care and saving money.) Once COVID-19 led to mass cancellations of in-person visits, it made the need for alternatives both immediate and undeniable. Soon came an emergency declaration expanding Medicare and Medicaid's reimbursement for telehealth services; the U.S. Food and Drug Administration also relaxed its rules for remote monitoring devices.[443] Private health insurers have followed this expansion of benefits to some extent.

Previously, only a small percentage of persons had ever experienced a remote virtual care visit. Over a matter of weeks, the number was 25 to 50 percent of patients, i.e., 50 to 175 *times* more patients seen via telemedicine than prepandemic. The key changes responsible for this shift were parity in payment for video visits, allowing patients' homes to serve as spoke sites, not requiring a prior patient-provider relationship, waiving of co-payments and deductibles and allowing doctors to practice across state lines.[444] It had already been estimated that $250 billion in annual costs could be saved by *virtualizing* parts of health care as now practiced, i.e., using telemedicine for just one fifth of emergency department care and one fourth of office visits.[445] Now over half of surveyed physicians plan to increase use of telemedicine in their practices. But despite patients' and providers' positive responses, all temporary rules may not remain in place after pandemic-related issues have subsided. CMS has permanently raised telemedicine reimbursement rates for rural areas and, not to worry, is commissioning more studies. Unfortunately, it takes Congressional action to continue payment for urban telemedicine and at-home visits in both settings.[446] Oh, brilliant.

Nearly half of U.S. hospitals with ICU beds do not have an intensivist on staff.[447] To the rescue comes *tele-ICU*, or *e-ICU*. Doctors first used remote viewing of intensive care patients nearly 50 years ago. It's now estimated more than one fourth of all hospital ICU units and almost one fifth of all ICU beds in the United States are supervised by remote providers from about 50 e-ICU hubs located throughout the nation. Each serves 50 to 500 patients using the *bunker model,* a bank of video monitors accompanied by the observer's full access to medical telemetry. The remote physician observes and evaluates, adjusts medical equipment settings, orders tests and medications and consults with bedside providers. On-site health care workers are intensivists or specially trained ICU RNs, NPs or PAs, and remote care can be administered from within the same medical complex or from another continent.

When the ability to diagnose, observe and treat is only a computer screen away, there are no geographic restrictions on a clinician's patient panel or a facility's constituency. However, there continue to be inherent limitations. None of these telemedicine advancements amount to much if the provider and patient don't have sufficient broadband internet service, hardware or the skills needed to effectively use them. COVID-19 demonstrated the many false assumptions and assertions previously made about providers' ability to offer and patients' ability to access health care technology. Forty percent of Americans don't have broadband in the home; access is low for racial minorities and those with less education and income; only about half of seniors have a smartphone suitable for teleconferencing and more than one fourth don't even use the Internet.[448] As we discovered, scheduling virtual care and vaccination appointments (and K-12 online schooling) entailed insurmountable challenges for many cohorts in many geographic areas. The Federal Communications Commission (FCC) claims only 21 million Americans are unserved by high speed broadband, but private entities put numbers at 25 to 50 percent of the total population. That leaves between 42 and 163 million Americans without internet service adequate for telemedicine and other telehealth monitoring services, and they don't all live in rural America. Maybe an agenda item for one of the FCC's 22 advisory committees . . .[449]

Besides the potential savings in personnel costs, it's also great to think telemedicine might reduce transfers out of small or remote hospitals and allow otherwise understaffed facilities to provide needed emergency, acute and chronic care management. Will an industry still unprepared to fully implement telemedicine commit to needed adjustments so remote health care can reach its full potential? It's clear telemedicine's highest and best use won't be realized until logistics are easy to implement and navigate for patients—and profitable for providers. Health care personnel and patients need effective guidance on how best to facilitate a virtual care consultation. System-wide issues concerning internet access, privacy, patient preparation and compliance with aftercare instructions must be addressed.[450] Let's hope that happens, because taking full advantage of telemedicine's benefits may ultimately do more than just reduce patient care costs and physician burnout. It may also provide better health outcomes.[451]

Strategies for self-preservation / Telemedicine

Telemedicine is another tool for delivering the best health care has to offer, including services not otherwise available at the patient's location. The use of remote clinicians can potentially address challenges of transportation, lack of mobility, time away from work and *white coat syndrome* (anxiety caused by being in a doctor's office). Telemedicine has proven advantages in the management of chronic illness and it may even solve some of the labor shortages we're facing. But as is true with much of health care technology, it is not without its drawbacks. There are obvious limitations for a provider who is able to use only two of the five senses in examining a patient. If some variation of virtual care sounds like it might benefit you or a loved one, learn about its availability and advisability for the health care situation at hand. Then seek your provider's guidance on the role and responsibilities for the patient—or the advocate/caregiver—in making it happen. What hardware and software does it require? How should the patient dress for a remote exam? Do cybersecurity threats increase when telemedicine apps are introduced into the patient's technology?

Here are hints for making the most of remote care and getting up to speed on your role in having a positive and effective telemedicine experience:

- For telemedicine in a hospital setting, verify if you or your loved one will be monitored by a remote hospitalist or intensivist because 1) you should always know who is providing care, no matter where they're located, and 2) it may impact the manner and timing of provider-patient-proxy communications.
- At home, ask your provider for written information on what you will need for cellphone or computer capacity and equipment, such as a microphone and camera.
- Clearly understand how the telemedicine connection is made and whether you need to install an app ahead of time on the smartphone or computer.
- Verify the time and date of your telemedicine visit and whether there is a pre-appointment log-in procedure.
- Find a private, quiet and well-lit location to use your phone or locate your tablet, laptop or desktop computer.
- If you need an interpreter or *appointment buddy* to assist with technology or to take notes, make those arrangements well ahead of time.
- Prior to the appointment, learn how to adjust the camera and volume so you can see and hear, as well as be seen and be heard.
- Have your medical history, medication list, notes on symptoms and any recent vitals, such as weight and temperature, close by. Have a list at hand of all doctors you are currently seeing and your calendar to refer to for recent events or new appointments.
- Make sure the computer is plugged in or fully charged and it's best to have other background apps closed to make the most efficient use of the telemedicine app.
- The doctor may be running late, so be patient at the appointed time—you'll be grateful if *your* appointment runs long. Know how to contact the provider's office for assistance if there's a technology glitch before or during the appointment.
- Arrange for someone to take notes or ask the doctor's permission to record the virtual care session on your smartphone for reference later. Keep a pad of paper and pen handy for notetaking and test any recording device ahead of time.

- Wear loose or appropriate clothing that's easy to remove if you need to display any part of your body during the appointment.
- Just as in a face-to-face appointment, don't part company without knowing the next step for diagnosis or treatment and who is responsible for making it happen.

And don't take the dog for walkies just before your telemedicine appointment is scheduled to begin. I'm serious. Do not do it.

Technology in diagnostics and treatment

Some diagnostics and treatments are possible and available for the first time thanks to technology, and it's posed to make others more accurate and reliable than ever before. Here are a few of many techie options already available and in development:

- Artificial intelligence, or *deep learning*, used by radiologists and pathologists to evaluate radiology tests.
- Blood sugar levels measured using a monitor that dispenses insulin as needed.
- Ingestible pill cams (*edible electronics*) swallowed by a patient to transmit raw video from throughout the digestive system.
- The logistics of a complex surgical procedure preplanned by previewing a patient's organs duplicated on a 3D printer or using virtual reality.
- Robotic surgery performed by a surgeon from another location or with a remote-controlled mini-robot (a *nanobot*) guided through the body.
- Incisions made with an intelligent surgical scalpel using smart sensor technology to identify malignant tissue for removal.
- A unique pharmacotherapy treatment plan created using pharmacogenomics to evaluate a patient's genetics.
- Laparoscopic surgery performed through minimally invasive incisions, which reduces healing time and the occurrence of surgery site infections.
- Artificial organs, joints, implants and bones produced by 3D printers.
- Low levels of electrical current used by brain stimulation devices to treat depression.
- Susceptibility to life-limiting diseases predicted with genetic testing, for use in family planning or preventive care.[452]

There's no question that for anyone working hard to be a fully engaged and informed decision maker, the presence of technology both complements and complicates that process. As we've progressed from waiting while X-ray film is developed to real-time digital radiography, our role in decision making has not diminished. Being fully engaged is still pivotal to having the right diagnostics done by the right people, and using that input to make an informed and comprehensive treatment plan.

Telemedicine has applications far beyond "*Do I have CoVid or not?*" and "*What the hell is this thing, doc?*" Health care kiosks reminiscent of a 1960s photo booth on steroids can turn any public space or waiting room into a clinic. Connected to a remote provider, the kiosk's audio and video technology may also include a stethoscope, EKG, thermometer, pulse oximeter and an automated pharmacy to dispense common medications. These free-standing step-in cubicles can even be a means of delivering mental health therapy.[453] Using *telestroke* technology to remotely observe a person in real time, a neurologist can evaluate a patient in an ambulance, care for someone in the ED of a remote rural hospital or check on an ICU patient.[454]

Try this one on. In 2014, Congress passed the *Protecting Access to Medicare Act* requiring the use of *artificial intelligence* (AI) for the preapproval of certain advanced diagnostic tests. Think a CT scan, X-ray, ultrasound, PET scan or MRI and think for heart disease, back pain, lung cancer or a suspected blood clot. In general, AI means using the formulas and algorithms of computer software, rather than the human brain, to make health care decisions. Under this new Medicare rule, the choice will be whether the patient qualifies to have certain diagnostic tests. Providers who fail to participate will risk not being paid.[455] Private organizations are developing the appropriate use criteria (AUC) and algorithm software to merge the AUC for each procedure with the patient's EHR—yup, the same ones now lacking both accuracy and interoperability—using an approved Clinical Decision Support Mechanism (CDSM). That will determine the medical suitability of the procedure for the specific patient. The provider will either get authorization for Medicare payment—or not. Full implementation has been delayed several times and is now scheduled to begin January 1, 2022.[456] At some point after Medicare starts using this AI process for some beneficiaries, expect private insurers to follow suit. Anyway, it's quite a shift in decision making authority. Honestly, there are so many ways for this to go wrong, I hardly know where to begin, but see *Self-preservation Strategies* / ***Diagnostics & treatment*** below for guidance on maintaining advocacy and safety.

Technological advances in the diagnosis and treatment of medical conditions are coming at us fast and furious—the choices are dizzying. It soon becomes tempting to accede to the wisdom of health care providers and abdicate all decision-making responsibility. Don't. This is when *knowing what you don't know* comes in really handy.

Strategies for self-preservation / Diagnostics & treatment

More options for diagnosing and then treating our medical conditions naturally require more decision making and a greater burden of accountability for both patient and provider. For health care consumers, there is no reasonable expectation of expertise, other than learning enough to make fully informed decisions and safely manage care. The crucial first step in that process of achieving optimal health outcomes is almost always getting a timely and accurate diagnosis. So, before we move on to the subject of seeking a second opinion, it's prudent to cover the basics of a *first* opinion.

The protocol for getting timely and accurate answers doesn't change when technology is introduced. Of course, my providers know I will follow the discovery of every disconcerting symptom with a search on the Internet, so they're not surprised when I arrive with my own theory of what's going on and what's to be done about it. But I'm definitely there to seek their medical expertise, so I'm as specific as possible about the issue's history and how it manifests itself. Like taking the car into the shop, the more symptoms and funny sounds I can describe, the more likely we'll figure out what's wrong. But no matter how long or how well your doctor knows you, it's unfair to assume total recall.

- Refresh your doctor's memory about previous or current medical conditions that are possibly relevant. Ask the provider to check that data against your EHR.
- If you're not asked, volunteer information on any medications you're taking or recent changes in their usage or side effects. Since you don't know for sure what the doctor sees in your EHR, it's another opportunity to verify accuracy.
- Whether the plan is for a test, procedure, medication, moving on to a specialist or watchful waiting, it should always be preceded by shared decision making, from disclosure and discussion through consent.
- Once you and the doctor agree on the next step or a treatment plan, it falls on you to follow up as needed or to report on new symptoms or unexpected changes.

I have always believed in the adage: *If you don't know what you're doing, surround yourself with those who do.* When an innovative test, procedure or therapy regimen is suggested, it's perfectly fine to ask your physician how long it's been in use, their personal observations and experience with it, what's known about the overall success rate and what premarket testing has been done. Medical devices do not require the same regulatory scrutiny as new drugs, so don't assume there have been numerous or long-term tests simply because a technology has FDA approval and is available.[457] When is a techie treatment or device no longer *experimental* and advisable for you?

- How many patients over what test period have been successfully treated?
- How does your health care situation factor into recommended applications?
- For procedures not fully vetted, is this the only available option?
- What is the advisability of doing nothing? Of *watchful waiting*?

The answers to these questions will be as unique as you, your medical history and your current condition. In any event, doing your own independent medical research on potential risks and outcomes is in order, no matter how long a device or procedure has been around. Once you and your provider make a shared decision on how to proceed, learn about your role in the treatment plan. The most up-to-date technology, such as a glucose monitor or automated medication dispenser, is of little value if not properly set up, used and maintained by the patient.

It's well-established that some medical procedures already require an insurer's preapproval, but with the upcoming CMS use of artificial intelligence, it's more important than ever for medical records to be complete and accurate. If your doctor recommends a diagnostic test or procedure and approval is denied, put on your advocate's hat and start asking questions. Garbage in/garbage out, as they say. Whether it's artificial intelligence or a human underwriter, only information provided can be processed. What is the evidentiary basis for denial? Is it founded on accurate data about your medical history, symptoms and personal information? Does medical research support approval, based on your situation? If you're engaged and trust your doctor, this is the occasion to join forces to achieve the best possible health outcomes.

There are times when it's appropriate to seek a second opinion and, to repeat, here they are:

- If the condition or treatment has life-threatening risks.
- If the diagnosis is uncertain.
- If the treatment is experimental.
- If required by insurance.
- If you get a funny feeling at the back of your head.

I've already covered the precautions for transferring medical records from one provider to another. Part of that recommended oversight is because it's so important that a diagnostician work from accurate and comprehensive test results. Once you've verified the second opinion provider has received all relevant EHRs, follow up with questions to make sure the second opinion is based on valid, complete and up-to-date information about you, your medical history and your present condition.

Strategies for self-preservation / Technology & medical errors

After reading the past few chapters, you can see that health care technology is loaded with potential for medical errors. Those are the hazards that come with enhancements. With all its treatments and cures undreamt of not long ago, technology does present new risks for adverse events. Your awareness can reduce or even eliminate many of them. *Ever vigilant.*

- *Electronic Health Records.* Mistakes in a patient's health care data can lead to medical errors concerning medications, diagnoses or treatments. Oversee the contents of your EHRs, such as medical history, current issues or precautions, allergies and medical devices, for inclusion and accuracy—and insist on corrections.
- *The lack of interoperability.* The inability to seamlessly access and transfer EHRs between providers can leave you with insufficient or no existing medical records in

an emergency or when you visit a new provider, a specialist or seek a second opinion. When possible, determine ahead of time the level of interoperability and always keep your own record of medical highlights available.

- *Patient matching in Electronic Health Records.* These hazards are all too common. Do not assume it's *your* complete and accurate EHR being accessed while you receive health care. Do not assume a treatment, procedure or medication is meant for you. Do not assume.
- *Remote patient monitoring and wearables.* As a tool for acute or chronic care management, telehealth is invaluable but never an unequivocal replacement for humans, i.e., you and your doctor. Telehealth monitoring is as reliable as its technology and the input data—and the humans utilizing its output. It cannot be an excuse to be less than fully aware of and informed about care management.
- *Internet health care resources.* When visiting websites to check symptoms or research treatment options, keep in mind they are only information-gathering conveniences, and not personalized opinions from trained medical professionals. If you rely on technology such as a smartphone app as a record of your vital health care data and interactions, maintain its accuracy so it doesn't become a source of misinformation in an emergency.
- *Medical devices.* Become familiar with precautions accompanying any hardware you are fitted with, such as a pacemaker or insulin monitor. Understand the meaning of alerts and appreciate the risks of interaction with other medical devices, diagnostic tests, medications or the activities of everyday life.
- *Telemedicine.* Remote clinical appointments can be both cost and time saving for providers and patients, but they impede visible clues that can be overlooked without a face-to-face examination. Incomplete information can lead to a misdiagnosis. First consider whether telemedicine is appropriate for your circumstances and whether your medical issue would be best evaluated in person. If proceeding with virtual care is the best choice, accept the duties that accompany your role in making it an effective alternative.

Want to make your computer go really fast? Throw it out the window. Most of us have a love-hate relationship with information technology. It's no different in the health care arena: Technology can be life-saving, a source of harm or a plain old pain in the neck. Learn to make peace with this frienemy. As a member of your health care team, it is here to stay.

CHAPTER FIFTEEN

Medication and polypharmacy

Few qualities of medicine are as amazing as the ability to use a vaccine for cancer prevention or a single pill to treat cardiovascular disease. Modern pharmaceuticals confer awesome powers of healing and disease management, but with them come serious responsibilities. It's time we gave pharmacotherapy the respect it deserves.

One pill, two pill, red pill, blue pill

Medication is an essential part of health care we have come to know and love—and, admittedly, take for granted. Maintenance drugs address chronic conditions, such as hypertension, heart disease and diabetes; specialty drugs are there for life-limiting or complex illnesses, e.g., cancer or Parkinson's; we rely on antibiotics and pain relievers for an acute infection or injury; and even emergency care has its clot-busters and drugs to reverse an opioid overdose. As you focus on achieving the best possible health outcomes for yourself and others, pharmaceuticals are not to be ignored as a potential source of medical misadventure. Imagine losing your independence simply because the side effects of a drug were mistaken for the onset of dementia. It could happen.

Almost six billion prescriptions were filled in America in 2018, enough to give 17.6 to each man, woman and child. Yowza. We spend about $370 billion each year on prescribed medicine in America, which is projected to reach $405 billion to $435 billion by 2023. The most popular prescriptions among all adults are for the chronic conditions of depression, high cholesterol, diabetes and heart disease.[458]

Keeping in mind what you now know about health care in America, this data should come as no surprise:

- One third of those aged 18 to 44 take at least one prescription each day.
- Two thirds of all prescriptions address chronic medical conditions.[459]
- Eighty percent of seniors are taking two or more prescriptions.
- Over one third of older adults take five or more prescriptions, which is how *polypharmacy* is defined.[460]
- About one fifth of those aged 65 and older take ten or more drugs.[461]

Before I get into specifics on how to aim for the best health outcomes in pharmacotherapy, let's cover the definitions relating to its darker side:

- A *medication error* is a mistake leading to inappropriate medication use or patient harm. It can occur anywhere in the process, from placing and executing the prescription order to dosing the drug to failing to monitor compliance; and it can be an error of either commission or omission. When the mistake causes patient harm, it is an *adverse drug event*. Medication errors cause an estimated 7,000 to 9,000 deaths each year in the United States, and the otherwise unnecessary health care expenses of morbidity and mortality (medical conditions and death) resulting from medication errors are estimated at $600 billion a year.[462]
- *Adverse drug events* (ADEs) are injuries resulting from medical intervention in any way related to a drug. They include medication errors, as well as adverse drug reactions, unintended and harmful drug interactions and overdoses. Annually, adverse drug events account for more than 3.5 million office visits, approximately one million trips to the emergency room and about 125,000 hospital admissions, along with negatively impacting two million hospitalizations.[463] The likelihood of polypharmacy goes up with age, and the risk of an ADE goes up with polypharmacy.[464] Among the most common ADEs in older adults are falls, Parkinsonism, kidney impairment, delirium, depression, sedation and low blood pressure. Oh, and according to HHS, about half of ADEs are preventable.[465]
- *Adverse drug reactions* (ADRs) are a subcategory of ADEs where there is a direct causal relationship between taking the drug and the harmful outcome. These allergic reactions can be as benign as a rash or as deadly as anaphylactic shock. Some are preventable errors, such as giving a drug to someone with a known allergy or failing to check for potentially dangerous drug-drug interactions. Many are not, as when an allergy is previously unknown or develops over time. Preventable or otherwise, the 2.2 million ADRs occurring each year in hospitalized patients cause over 106,000 deaths. To be clear, an adverse drug reaction is *not* the same as an unintended and negative side effect of a medication.[466]

I'll wager all these numbers will be going up, not down, over the coming years, which will mean more potential for harmful outcomes and increased health care utilization and costs.

The very beginning of the prescribing process, whether it's the ordering of a drug or failing to do so, accounts for almost half of all medication errors. It may be a lack of familiarity with the patient's medical or medication history, distractions, EHR inaccuracies, technology failures, poor penmanship (old school), mouse-clicking the wrong medication (new school) or ordinary incompetence.[467] Whatever the source or specifics of a medication error, the effect can be life-altering, e.g., the patient's death when excessive blood thinner causes a brain bleed or less visible harm, when an improperly used antibiotic provides no therapeutic benefit.[468]

Patient autonomy remains a significant factor when it comes to the effective use of medications. How each one of us affects the drugs we take is *pharmacokinetics,* and how drugs we take affect each one of us is *pharmacodynamics*. Any medication can have exceptional consequences in the youngest and oldest among us because age and body mass impact how humans absorb, distribute, metabolize and eliminate drugs. That's important to bear in mind with a new prescription, as well as in managing a chronic condition over time. Even though polypharmacy is present in 36 to 40 percent of those aged 65 and older, clinical drug trials often underrepresent the geriatric crowd, even when they will be the ultimate users of the medicine being tested. Doing so ignores vital information about the effectiveness and side effects of certain drugs in older patients and potentially adds to ADEs in seniors due to a lack of valid drug precautions.[469]

Because it involves *medications associated with geriatric syndromes* (MAGS), polypharmacy in the elderly brings the additional risks of delirium, cognitive impairment, falls, reduced appetite or weight loss, incontinence and depression. For example, one of the most popular MAGS, antidepressants, can cause five out of six geriatric syndromes—in fact, every one except depression.[470] When patients are discharged from the hospital to skilled nursing with an average of 14 prescriptions in tow, it's little wonder risks for unintended harm are present. Adverse interactions and side effects explain how someone not otherwise cognitively impaired ends up in a memory unit. Pharmacotherapy is complicated business.

Here are the most common causes of adverse drug events. For the record, any one of them can trigger an ADE for a health care consumer of any age, and they are *not* in order of incidence because those statistics don't exist:

- Patient mismatching causes the records of the wrong patient to be accessed.
- Reliance on incomplete or erroneous medical records.
- A lack of knowledge about the patient's medical or medication history.
- The failure to fully understand the patient's current medical condition.
- Prescribing a drug without first examining the patient.
- A prescription given in the absence of any medical indication.
- A provider's inadequate knowledge of a drug's appropriate use.
- The overuse of a drug due to an erroneous dosage or patient misuse.
- The failure to prescribe a drug appropriate for the patient's condition.
- Human error in placing an electronic order without proper safety measures.
- A provider's inadequate knowledge of a drug's contraindications and side effects.
- Poorly labeled consumer drugs that contribute to confusion or misreadings.
- Labels or abbreviations in automated dispensers that invite human error.
- Look-alike labeling or packaging of drugs used in a hospital or care facility.

- A technology failure in an ordering system without proper safety measures.
- Failure to note a patient's drug allergy in the medical record.
- A harmful interaction with another drug, food or medical test.
- Failure to have a patient's medications and symptoms regularly reviewed.
- A drug's side effect mistaken for the symptom of a medical condition.
- A consumer's misunderstanding about a drug's storage or dosage instructions.
- The unintentional skipping of a dose or taking extra doses.
- A technology failure in a remote system used to monitor or dispense drugs.
- A mistake in labeling a container's contents as to drug name or weight.
- The consumer skipping a dose because of drug costs or unpleasant side effects.
- Miscommunication between health care professionals.
- A consumer's lack of knowledge about and awareness of possible side effects.
- A provider mishearing a drug name or the misuse of drug abbreviations.
- Technology failures in the voice recognition of a provider's drug order.
- The use of multiple providers and/or pharmacies without any oversight.
- Miscommunication during a care handoff.

Whoa. If that seems like an alarming number of opportunities for a medication blunder to occur, it is. Reliable industry-wide statistics on the frequency and type of medication errors would help stakeholders, individual providers and patients to drill down more precisely on actionable preventive measures. However, as with medical errors of any type, there is no nationwide mandatory reporting system for medication errors. U.S. Food and Drug Administration data collection is voluntary, so it's difficult to draw conclusions, even from the 100,000 reports this agency does receive each year.[471] There may be limited value in knowing one private patient safety organization has calculated the proportion of medication errors within its own data and found 27 percent of medical errors were drug-related. Of those, more than two thirds were "wrong events": wrong dose, wrong patient or wrong administration of the drug.[472]

Now for the true story of someone whose life became a perfect storm of medication missteps. Sadly, similar scenarios materialize often enough to have their own label: a *prescribing cascade*. To begin with, this 71-year-old woman had high blood pressure, type 2 diabetes, asthma, hypothyroidism, depression, osteoarthritis and Meniere's disease, a disorder of the inner ear. In the United States, she would be among one in every ten seniors for this number of comorbidities. As if all that weren't enough for her to deal with, the real trouble began when . . .

- Her family physician prescribed a blood pressure medicine.
- Four months later, she developed edema (swelling) of the legs, so her cardiologist put her on two diuretics to flush excess fluids.

- Three weeks passed and her urologist gave her another prescription to treat the symptoms of an apparent overactive bladder.
- Her family physician ordered a new medicine thirty days later to relieve the dry mouth she complained of.
- One month after that, she fell in her bathroom, injuring her head and back. She ended up in the ED with severe pain from multiple fractures.
- When she arrived, she was on 17 different medications.

Once hospitalized, she was seen by a clinical pharmacist who—lucky for the patient—recognized the unmistakable signs of a prescribing cascade. He also noted at least five of her medications had increased the risk of her having a fall. A geriatrician *deprescribed* (yes, that's a word) the five most recent prescriptions and put her on a blood pressure medication without edema as a side effect. The patient was hospitalized for 14 days, stabilized and then released to a rehab center.

The geriatric hospitalist tracked the trail of medication bloopers that had ultimately harmed this patient and led to her hospitalization. Beginning with the cardiologist, every doctor had mistakenly interpreted a drug side effect as the symptom of a new medical issue. Consistently, the response of each had been to prescribe an additional drug, causing more adverse drug events.[473] And so on and so forth.

Much like our subject here, the most likely victims of a prescribing cascade have a complex medical story, multiple prescribers, use more than one pharmacy, fail to have regular reviews of all medications and suffer from poor—or no—communication between providers.[474] This ill-fated lady unwittingly became the poster child for medication errors:

- ✓ The failure to fully understand the patient's current medical condition.
- ✓ Reliance on incomplete or erroneous medical records.
- ✓ A lack of knowledge about the patient's medical or medication history.
- ✓ A provider's inadequate knowledge of a drug's contraindications and side effects.
- ✓ A drug's side effect mistaken for the symptom of a medical condition.
- ✓ The failure to prescribe a drug appropriate for the patient's condition.
- ✓ The use of multiple providers and/or pharmacies without any oversight.
- ✓ Failure to have a patient's medications and symptoms regularly reviewed.
- ✓ Miscommunication between health care professionals.
- ✓ A consumer's lack of knowledge about and awareness of possible side effects.

There were several missed opportunities to avoid this prescribing cascade or at least to detect it, had any one of her several providers widened their gaze even a little. Apparently, in order to be safe, this is what it has come to: Any new symptom should be assumed to be medication-related until there is solid evidence of another cause for the patient's symptoms. The upside is that nearly all the systemic and individual failures that befell this 71-year-old lady, and could just as easily happen to one of us, are also entirely preventable.

Strategies for self-preservation / Medication & polypharmacy

Before even one preventive action step is taken, it's crucial to acknowledge that medication deserves the same level of shared decision making as any other proposed medical treatment. After full disclosure and discussion of the patient's autonomous perspective, the medical reason for the proposed pharmacotherapy, all available options and their risks and benefits, it's time to ask, "*Considering all personal and treatment goals, is this the right thing to do?*"

In preparing to have that discussion, the doctor needs complete and up-to-date records on all existing symptoms, conditions, medications and history. Based on what you've learned about EHRs, you recognize your responsibility to verify or correct what the provider is seeing on the computer screen and to make amendments or addendums as needed. In the case of multiple physicians located in more than one facility—or even more than one department—it's a virtual certainty your medical records will not be complete and fully accurate without some help from you.

As patient or advocate, please be fully forthcoming about symptoms, no matter how embarrassing or inconsequential they may seem. The clinician relies on those clues to accurately diagnose medical needs. I'm a big fan of what I call a **Good-To-Meet-You-&-In-Case-of-Emergency Profile**, either in writing or on a smartphone app, containing highlights of the patient's complete medical story. (It's also a must-have in case you visit a new provider or in an emergency.) And yes, that means either the patient or the advocate needs to be familiar with every medication and why it was prescribed.

Giving consent for a new prescription is not the end of the shared decision making process. A full discussion of dosage instructions, potential side effects and when they might be cause for concern should follow the decision to begin a new drug.

- *Does "Take three daily" mean all at once or spread throughout the day?*
- *Should dosing be coordinated with eating?*
- *Are there foods or beverages to be avoided?*
- *Does this drug get along with other medications you're already taking?*
- *How will you know if it's working?*
- *Do you need to finish the prescription if symptoms go away?*
- *What's the next step when the drug protocol is finished? Is it ever finished?*

Anytime you fill a prescription, read the container label to confirm its contents agree with your understanding and/or with previous refills. If you have a question, the pharmacist is right there. And check the label every time you dispense the drug, whether into a pill minder or into your mouth.

Are health care consumers properly storing most drugs? Sure, if *dry* and *cool* describe the bathroom and the window sill in the kitchen. Not. Ask for the pharmacist's recommendation. Speaking of pharmacies, you should have only one if possible. More in the next chapter about care management, but having a designated provider or pharmacist to watch out for potential drug interactions or contraindications takes you one step closer to medication safety. Little stuff matters, like:

- The *tablespoon* for meds is not the same as the one for ice cream.
- It is not okay to chew a nonchewable.
- Splitting a pill is only safe if the pharmacist or doctor says it is.
- Confusing eardrops and eyedrops should be avoided.
- If you have a major pill spill, let the pharmacist sort them out.[475]

Consider taking all your drugs for an outing. It's referred to as a *medication reconciliation*, also known as a *Brown Bag Checkup*. Medicare calls it a *Medication Therapy Management Program*. You tote all those bottles to your pharmacist or primary care provider for a comprehensive review—and toss in over-the-counter meds, vitamins and herbal supplements while you're at it. Research shows these assessments, followed by necessary deprescribing interventions, can result in a 59 percent reduction in patients with potentially inappropriate meds, a 24 percent reduction in the number of fallers and a 26 percent reduction in mortality.[476] If your provider doesn't regularly include a med review in visits, use your annual checkup or wellness review to verify bottles against your medical records, including why and how each medication should be taken versus reality. For the record, it doesn't do any good to be less than forthright about how and when you take each drug, including overuse, inconsistent use or nonuse.

Pills have become such an accepted part of our health care journey, it's sometimes easy to forget the vital role they play in achieving the best health outcomes and the punch those tiny little guys can deliver. You're about to learn about an important step in every health care journey, and it's another time when pharmacotherapy often fails to gets the respect it deserves.

CHAPTER SIXTEEN

Care management and handoffs

Gone are the days of the long-term and monogamous doctor-patient relationship. With comorbidities, specialists, levels of care, complex pharmacotherapy and sophisticated rehabilitation, consistent oversight is key to safety and achieving the best health outcomes. Otherwise, there can be dangerous and unintended consequences.

It's time for *somebody* to be in charge

There's a process for staying as safe as possible while receiving the most competent and appropriate health care. It's called *care management*, a patient-centered method of coordinating care for those with one or more chronic medical conditions or complex needs. Medicare's care management benefit requires the patient to have at least two chronic health conditions, but some level of care management is appropriate for a patient of any age who sees more than one provider and/or is being discharged from one level of care to another, which is a *care handoff*.

If you think of health care as a team activity, care management defines the role of the coach, a role that's usually filled by a primary care provider (PCP), the attending hospital physician or a specialist. The goal is to help the patient better understand health issues and achieve the best health outcomes with the most effective and safe delivery of care. The care coordinator's duties are performed outside regular doctor visits. They include referrals to specialists and ancillary services; coordination of all providers; medication management; oversight of tests and procedures; and support of patient compliance, healthy living and self-care. Before considering how care management is instrumental in achieving the best health outcomes throughout a health care journey, let's first fully understand what we hope to gain.

Just when you thought it was safe . . .

If asked to name the most dangerous time in a health care journey, most would guess it's during a major surgery or risky test or maybe in the midst of a *code blue,* when everyone is rushing to save your life. Nope. The most dangerous time is not even while actively undergoing a medical treatment or procedure. It's during *care handoffs*, when you're simply being moved from one level of care to another or being transferred between providers.[477] These are the most common care transitions:

- Being treated by an unfamiliar clinician if your doctor is unavailable.
- Seeing a provider after being screened by a nurse in the exam room.
- Visiting a specialist on the recommendation of your PCP.
- Entering the ED after receiving care in an ambulance.
- Transferring from the ED to a hospital room or ICU.
- Going from postoperative recovery to a hospital room or ICU.
- Receiving care from new providers after a shift change or staff rotation.
- Being discharged from the hospital to rehab or home aftercare.

A handoff is the opportunity for meaningful communication between the giver and receiver of patient information, which means it is also ripe for failure.[478] Think about it. When someone is transported to the hospital by ambulance, there can be as many as seven handoffs involving vital information and/or the patient. The actors involved include the 911 caller; emergency dispatcher; paramedics; patient; family or friends of the patient; emergency department dispatcher; and, finally, ED health care professionals. An omission or misunderstanding anywhere along this communication chain can trigger a life-or-death outcome.[479] Risks are similar when going from the ED to hospital admission and from there to a care center or home. Consider all the critical medical info that should be exchanged between providers and caregivers for the next level of care to go well. It's a lot, and just one disregarded instruction can cause an adverse event or a missed follow-up appointment or an otherwise unnecessary hospital readmission.

Then there's the autonomous and personal information that providers and caregivers need to know, such as usual living arrangements, family situation, existing comorbidities, medications, allergies, care preferences, personality traits, mobility challenges, impairments and cognitive issues. Is it even possible to remain safe as a patient unless everyone in your chain of care knows your story? Threats to safety, invisibility, electronic health records, medications and care handoffs. The elements of health care hazardous to patient autonomy and safety are perilously intertwined.

What do we know about how a badly executed handoff can impact inpatient and aftercare? Studies show:

- One third of older women diagnosed with a fragility bone fracture are not instructed to follow up with osteoporosis screening after injury.[480]
- More than two thirds of patients have an error in their medication history during hospital admission that continues through time of discharge.[481]
- While hospitalized, almost half of patients going from the ICU to a regular hospital room experience a medication error during transfer.[482]
- A move from the hospital back to a nursing home involves an adverse event for nearly half of all discharges, with 70 percent found to be preventable.[483]

It's not that we lack the tools for safe and productive handoffs, we just aren't using them. Although both medical students and practicing clinicians agree more handoff training and implementation is needed and wanted, there are little, if any, standardized procedures in place during a doctor's classroom or clinical education.[484] The *I-PASS Handoff Bundle* is one example of many mnemonics available to guide the delivery of vital info along with patient care between shifts. When used, it shows a 23 percent reduction in medical errors and a 30 percent reduction in adverse events.[485] And the practice of including the patient's PCP in communication from the time of hospital admission through discharge and aftercare is a simple but effective application of coordinated and managed care.[486]

Naturally, there are financial considerations. While some care management interventions do have up-front operating and labor expenses for providers and facilities, a patient's total care costs are lowered if we take the time for effective communication. Yes, reducing emergency visits and otherwise unnecessary readmissions lowers expenditures.[487] Who knew? As for the value of preventing adverse events that potentially harm or kill patients? Priceless.

Home sweet medical home

A model of care that employs tools of coordination and communication for optimal care management is the *patient-centered medical home* (PCMH). This is a care philosophy, not a place. If you've heard of *fee-based* versus *value-based* payment models, the medical home is on the value-based side. It's a team approach coordinating all levels of care and involving the patient or proxy in decision making, whether it's about treatment for an acute illness, hospitalization, caregiving, rehab, socialization, nutrition, healthy living or chronic disease oversight—or handoffs between those levels of care. Instead of being a curse, technology is used for data and care management to monitor health, promote patient safety and facilitate the best possible health care. The patient-centered medical home reduces emergency care and hospital readmissions and enhances the patient-provider relationship while respecting patients' autonomous goals and preferences.[488]

This payment and care model has been around since 2007 and over the past decade has been widely tested by the federal government under various names, all designed to transform the industry from fee-for-service to pay-for-value.[489] Besides involving health care facilities and insurers, clinicians may even share in the financial rewards of having healthier clients. Sorry to report that only one in four doctors has implemented the Medicare chronic care management benefit, and it is used by less than ten percent of eligible beneficiaries. There is also Medicare's Transitional Care Management, which specifically addresses hazards in the hospital-to-home handoff. Its usage rate is as abysmal. Obstacles to implementation of this benefit include providers' low reimbursement rates, the burden of paperwork, the complexity of coding and the patient volume required to reach profitability. The last time someone had the stomach to measure the volume of Medicare and Medicaid regulations, there were 130,000 pages. That was over 20 years ago.[490]

Another of the federal government's own value-based models, Primary Cares Initiative, pays participating providers a monthly fee per patient, plus reimbursement for office visits.[491] Hey, that sounds a lot like the concierge and direct primary care models already being embraced by some practitioners. Granted, the CMS version is perhaps not quite as attractive, what with all the inherent government paperwork and regulations that concierge and DPC clinicians are trying to escape. Considering the nearly two-year delinquency in paying bonuses for CMS's Alternative Payment Model,[492] provider interest may wane. Time will tell if the government's versions of the PCMH are answers to the need for efficient and accessible health care resources.

Our expanding dependence on *hospitalists* may offer a path to care management, if properly executed. In fact, this care model offers PCMH-like care during hospitalization and might be a person's first experience with fully communicating health care team members. How does the handoff fit into this care management paradigm? If the PCP provides valuable context by telling the patient's medical story to the hospitalist upon admission, remains involved and in the communication chain throughout hospitalization and supports post-discharge treatment and caregiving goals, it creates a true care management model. Hazards of adverse events and readmissions inherent in care transitions are reduced as well. As for success in preventing the negative impact of adverse events, studies have shown:

- Implementing tools for communication during handoffs reduced the time it takes to transfer from the ED to a patient room by one third and resulted in a 50 percent decline in readmissions.[493]
- There is a significantly lower risk for hospital readmissions by having patients see their PCP for just 20 minutes within seven days of discharge.[494]
- The use of *patient navigators* for phone check-ins to schedule appointments and follow up with reminders reduced ED visits by 43 percent and readmissions by 58 percent.[495]
- Guidance in communication among families, nurses and physicians during pediatric hospital stays reduced preventable harmful adverse events by 38 percent, demonstrating the value in a *family-centered care model*.[496]

So many balls in the air. When a single doctor is treating several medical issues, an EHR contains errors or omissions and/or the doctor doesn't have the time to sufficiently review patient information, harmful conflicts can arise. Chronic conditions involving multiple specialists present similar safety risks involving drug interactions, duplication of services or medication side effects mistaken for symptoms.

By now you know how I feel about you being an engaged patient, but managing a medical condition on your own is beyond a health care consumer's level of expertise. That's the role of a health care *team* and is the intrinsic value in having one. Invite your primary care provider to be your care manager, and inform specialists to get communication and effective care management practices flowing in both directions.

Strategies for self-preservation / Care management & handoffs

You may or may not be surprised to learn nearly every tool developed until now to foster safer handoffs and care management—and there's a ton of them—was designed for use by providers, not health care consumers. And here's the other thing: There is *no question* that when handoffs are given the respect they deserve, patient falls, pressure injuries and medication errors are reduced. No question about that. Fine, if the health care industry isn't consistently sharing and facilitating standards for care management and handoffs, then it falls to each one of us to keep our health care journey as safe as possible. With preplanning and checklists at hand, we can be active comanagers of our care. Let's go back to the basics:

✓ ***First, you must be present to win.*** In the event you don't have the decision-making capacity to fully participate in managing your care—like, if you're having a health care crisis—while you *are* still fully capacitated, make a plan to always have an advocate present on your behalf.

✓ ***Second, care management—and most especially the handoff—requires shared decision making.*** Refer to Chapter Eleven for more detail, but the key steps are to fully consider the medical condition, the patient's autonomy, treatment options, all risks and benefits and the right to grant informed consent. Even as you are on your way out of the hospital, shared decision making is crucial to preserving patient safety.

✓ ***Third, verbal agreements are as good as the paper they're written on***, so insist that any handoff or aftercare instructions involving the patient or any member of their care team be in writing. Until we can guarantee every patient and provider full and functional access to reliable EHRs, the printed word still has a significant role in health care communications.

Establishing a medical home. Health care consumers who enjoy this approach to health care delivery are part of a cooperative health care team of patient, provider(s) and advocate or proxy decision maker. It promises much in overcoming the safety risks inherent in patient invisibility, medical errors, technology, medication, handoffs and care management. Even without a formal clinic-wide medical home care model, discuss having your PCP act as your trusted care manager, not just someone you see for an annual wellness visit or if you have an acute medical issue.

- Schedule a professional review of all medications and medical records on a periodic basis, including those maintained by independent specialists.
- When another provider suggests a test or procedure, consult with your PCP and seek counsel on advisability and any concerns you or they have.
- Encourage multiple providers to communicate with each other by asking that any changes in EHRs be made available to other members of your health care team.

Demonstrate being an empowered and engaged patient by encouraging all members of your team to cooperate in overseeing your health care and helping you achieve the best health outcomes.

Care level handoffs. For a handoff to be effective, there has to be one. It's more than just moving a patient from one level of care or from one provider to another. A real handoff is taking assertive steps to effectively pass on complete and accurate medical and personal information about the patient along with the person. The benchmark for success may be as complex as assembling a multi-disciplinary support team prior to the patient's transfer from hospital to hospice. Or it may be as simple as receiving an appointment reminder card at the end of each physical therapy session. As circumstances allow, make arrangements to have that crucial communication—no matter how elaborate or simple—anytime there's a care transition.

Handoff standards vary with the situation, but these suggestions for *health care professionals* apply anytime a patient transfers between levels of care or providers, whether seeing a specialist for the first time or going from the ambulance to the ED. It falls to the patient or advocate to urge compliance with this guidance:

- Determine the patient's capacity to participate in planning and decision making.
- Establish who the authorized decision maker will be, if the patient lacks capacity.
- Clearly identify who is managing the patient's care.
- If the answer is "*no one*," designate a professional or layperson as care manager.
- Learn and consider the patient's autonomous personal and treatment goals.
- Include the patient and any proxy decision maker in the planning process.
- Keep the patient or proxy informed of the patient's condition.
- Periodically review the patient's EHR for accuracy and completeness.
- Address any questions or concerns from the patient or advocate/proxy.
- Make clear any next steps, who should take them and when.

Hospital inpatient handoffs. During a hospital stay, you may be visited by a different PCP or specialist each day, depending on how hospital rounds are covered by providers. With the goal of maintaining consistent, effective and safe care, when there's a change in clinician and caregivers or a transfer from one level of care to another, communication between patient/advocate and health care professionals should include:

- The patient's identity, medical status and relevant personal story.
- The procedures and tests that have been done and are scheduled or anticipated.
- The patient's diagnosis, prognosis and treatment goals.
- The identity of all other providers and specialists attending the patient.
- The patient's advocate and/or proxy decision maker identity and contact info.

Two simple steps the advocate can take to facilitate an effective inpatient handoff are 1) to communicate directly with all providers prior to and after any transition and 2) to use the white board or a posted sign in the patient's room to identify the patient, important information concerning medical devices, allergies or dietary restrictions and the advocate's name and contact information.

Hospital discharge handoffs. When a patient is discharged from the hospital to another care setting or to home, the patient and advocate should seek clear communication with the discharge professional about:

- The reason for hospitalization and what tests and procedures were performed.
- The diagnosis and prognosis for the patient's current medical condition.
- A recommended treatment plan, including the use of any specialists.
- Follow-up appointments or treatments and who arranges for them.
- A list of medications stopped or begun during hospitalization.
- The purpose, dosage and potential adverse effects of any new medications.
- Caregiving needs and mobility challenges in the patient's daily living.
- Special equipment needs or recommended living arrangements.
- Cautions about side effects or symptoms to watch for and report.
- Communication protocols and contact information for all providers.
- The transfer of current medical records to other health care team members.
- Designation of who will act as the care manager or coordinator.
- Any prohibited or recommended activities.
- Special instructions, as for the use of monitoring devices or wound care.
- Detailed aftercare instructions and provider contact information *in writing*.

Throughout *Patient or Pawn?*, we have seen countless examples of how effective communication contributes to having the best health outcomes. Nowhere is it more palpable than in care management and care handoffs, which are both potential sources of patient harm. We cannot possibly reach the goal of having the best health outcomes through *patient-centered care* without also focusing on *team-centered care.*

Okay then.

A FEW CLOSING REMARKS

"Knowing is not enough; we must apply.
Willing is not enough; we must do."
- Johann Wolfgang von Goethe
Retooling for an Aging America:
Building the Health Care Workforce (2008)
Institute of Medicine of the National Academies

I discovered much of what you read in *Patient or Pawn?* just before you did, and I was no less astonished. We're in trouble, big, big trouble. Because of what happened 70 years ago when the United States had more births than ever before, we're now having more aging and aged than ever before. Not debatable. It doesn't help that nearly half of American adults of *all* ages have two or more chronic conditions. For every three of today's high-maintenance patients, there will be four or five by 2030. At the same time, for every three health care workers we'll need, there will only be two. All that is true, but none of it—or any other intervening health care crisis—diminishes the right you have to be informed and autonomous and safe while being cared for. And that remains true even if you lack decision making capacity and your advocate steps in.

What's coming is not a theoretical possibility. It is a no-kidding-people, this-is-happening impending crisis of demand versus supply. Perhaps there are lessons to be learned in what we've recently experienced. We should first acknowledge how eerily similar the elements of the pandemic were to the characteristics of the looming perfect storm: 1) Exceptionally large cohorts of high-maintenance aging and chronically ill patients, 2) a shortage of services and supplies to meet their demands and 3) consumers' lack of health literacy skills and reliable resources needed for informed care management. Maybe, just maybe, our health care leaders will use what we all witnessed to better anticipate and plan for the approaching threats relating to patient safety, invisibility, technology, medications, care management and handoffs. I hope so.

Because sick and dying people don't have the time, energy or resources to put up much of a fight, they find themselves low hanging fruit when policy makers and bureaucrats want to shift priorities. I'm beginning to think that might even be true for *people of a certain age*. Although the need for Medicare funding is projected to rise 8 percent every year going forward just to pace indisputable demographics, Medicare continues to remain a likely target when lawmakers and bureaucrats want to free up funds for other agendas.[497] That certainly works to boost seniors' popularity as patients. And since less than five percent of Americans live in nursing homes, it bears asking why those residents accounted for over one third of all COVID-19 deaths in the United

States.[498] Should we feign surprise? The federal ombudsmen program charged with protecting and advocating for disabled children and the elderly in America's care facilities is appallingly undervalued and underperforming—and always has been.[499] What I've seen and read has exposed systemic changes begging to be made:

- For crying out loud, would someone in a position of power puleez formulate some legitimate health care workforce projections? It escapes me why others aren't demanding this, like members of Congress, the COGME and every group alleging to advocate for providers or patients. It's almost like they don't want to know.
- The same goes for gathering and disseminating up-to-date and useable data on the hazards inherent in electronic health records, patient mismatching, harmful hospital-acquired conditions (32-year-old data), fatal falls (29-year-old data) and medical errors (really, no data). People should not be harmed or die solely as the result of being treated or hospitalized.
- The U.S. Department of Justice might consider updating its 2010 regulations for the *Americans With Disabilities Act*. Requiring only 2 percent of parking spaces to be handicapped-accessible when 19 percent of all American adults have issues with walking says a lot about a lot of things.[500]
- Huge segments of our country and its population face challenges of access to both health care *and* broadband service. Health care leaders need to either fund the nationwide upgrade to high-speed Internet service or start using existing capabilities for mobile health services and health care kiosks to overcome obvious inequities. For the homebound, areas with low provider ratios, impoverished neighborhoods, patients with infectious diseases . . .
- After 40 years of what should be crushing humiliation for its promoters, the *Healthy People* initiative needs to come off financial life support. Enough already. HHS might consider funding the promotion of preventive care at even a fraction of what it spends to measure irrelevant markers and treat avoidable medical conditions.
- The epidemic of chronic illness in America, including obesity and childhood diseases, is largely ignored as the health care crisis it truly is. We know how to prevent and manage this disaster, so why aren't we doing it?
- It's troubling to view the vagueness and denial that surround mental illness in America, visible both in bureaucrats' ignorance of its impact and in policy makers' refusal to provide comprehensive and equitable treatment. Shame on them.
- The recent $505 million HHS "health literacy" campaign "*to get these individual patients to make a different decision*" about COVID-19 vaccinations is a perversion of health literacy's true purpose: to preserve each person's right to give or withhold fully informed and autonomous consent.[501] The same goes for taxpayer-funded "vaccine lotteries." They are not promoting health literacy. Not even close.

- Let's pinpoint why the rate of fatal falls has risen so dramatically and implement plans for prevention—and let's do it pretty soon. HHS could start by updating the statistics it appears to be relying upon, nearly 30 years old.[502] Still not kidding.
- Why doesn't HHS or the American Medical Association or the American Pharmacists Association sponsor a *National Review of All Medications Week*? We know *Brown Bag Checkups* have measurable value because there is oodles of research showing the positive impact on both quality and quantity of life when we practice medication literacy. What's the holdup?

You know, if you or I had just one thin dime for every time we've heard a policy maker or bureaucrat use a term such as *urgent*, *not acceptable*, *immediate need* or *impending crisis*—only to discover 20 or 30 years later that they've made absolutely no progress. Well, we'd have a bunch of dimes. Every journey begins where we are and we find ourselves caught in the middle of a health care system where patient autonomy and safety are not valued priorities. Our access to timely and competent health care is in jeopardy as long as those controlling the resources don't make our best health outcomes the ultimate goal. So what's next? Where do we go from here?

- Form an organization to loudly advocate for America's most vulnerable health care consumers? *Maybe.*
- Do whatever it takes to fully appreciate our rights as patients and then work like hell to preserve them? *Most definitely.*
- Talk to the people we care about to make sure they know how precarious and hazardous a health care journey can be? *As soon and as often as possible.*

That's probably enough to get us started.

It was my intent to leave you with an awareness of the inevitable challenges faced by America's health care system and consumers, your rights as a patient and the available strategies for self-preservation. We can't change the system, but I hope you now see we have more control over individual health care experiences than one might think. Understand that even if you try to do everything I suggest, you won't always get it right the first time. I certainly don't. But I do what I can and I keep an eye on the end game of preserving rights to consent and autonomy and safety. Listen to the people you know you can trust and—as importantly—to the little voice at the back of your head.

I welcome hearing about the encounters along your health care journey, the scary parts as well as the times when patients and providers are wise and bold. You can reach me at *PatientOrPawn@outlook.com*. Oh, and tell your health care professionals how much you value them. They don't hear that nearly often enough.

Have a safe journey.

ENDNOTES

We really, really need a turtle crossing.
We have a lot of turtles in the road
and we're very worried about them.
- Anonymous

CHAPTER ONE

[1] Tony Leys, "Wrong cancer diagnosis leaves Iowan suffering after unnecessary surgery," Des Moines Register, January 3, 2019, www.dmregister.com; Ferdinando L. Mirarchi, DO, FAAEM, FACEP et al, "TRIAD I – The Realistic Interpretation of Advanced Directives," Journal of Patient Safety, December 2008, www.institutehcd.com; Ferdinando L. Mirarchi, DO, FAAEM, FACEP et al, "TRIAD II: Do Living Wills Have an Impact on Pre-hospital Lifesaving Care?," Journal of Emergency Medicine, January 21, 2009, American Academy of Emergency Medicine, www.institutehcd.com.

[2] French philosopher Auguste Comte, 1798 – 1857.

[3] Russell Heimlich, "Baby Boomers Retire," Pew Research Center FacTank, December 29, 2010, www.PewResearch.org.

[4] "2020 Alzheimer's Disease Facts and Figures," Alzheimer's & Dementia, Journal of the Alzheimer's Association, March 2020, Alzheimer's Association, www.alz.org.

[5] Peter I. Buerhaus, PhD et al, "Four Challenges Facing the Nursing Workforce in the United States," Journal of Nursing Regulation, July 2017, www.journalofnursingregulation.com.

CHAPTER TWO

[6] In the Matter of Karen Quinlan, an Alleged Incompetent, Supreme Court of New Jersey, 355 A.2nd 647 (New Jersey 1976).

[7] Nancy Beth Cruzan, By Her Parents and Co-Guardians, Lester L. Cruzan et ux. v. Director, Missouri Department of Health, et al, 497 U.S. 261 (1990).

[8] In re: Guardianship of Theresa Marie Schiavo, Incapacitated, Robert Schindler and Mary Schindler v. Michael Schiavo, as Guardian of the person of Theresa Marie Schiavo, In the District Court of Appeal of Florida Second District, Case No. 2D02-5394, June 6, 2003.

[9] Ravi Nessman, "Karen Ann Quinlan's Parents Reflect on Painful Decisions 20 Years Later," Los Angeles Times, April 7, 1996, www.latimes.com.

[10] Deaths and Death Rates for the 10 Leading Causes of Death, by Sex: United States, 1976, National Center for Health Statistics, accessed August 8, 2019, National Center for Health Statistics, Centers for Disease Control and Prevention, U.S. Department of Health and Human Services, www.cdc.gov/nchs.

[11] 10 Leading Causes of Death, United States / 2019 / All Races, Both Sexes, National Center for Injury Prevention and Control, National Center for Health Statistics, Centers for Disease Control and Prevention, February 20, 2020, U.S. Department of Health and Human Services, www.cdc.gov/nchs.

[12] "Hepatitis B - Yesterday, Today & Tomorrow: NIH Research Timelines," Research Portfolio Online Reporting Tools, National Institutes of Health, accessed October 30, 2019, U.S. Department of Health and Human Services, www.nih.gov.

[13] Deaths and Death Rates for Leading Causes of Death: Death Registration States, 1900-1940, National Vital Statistics System, National Center for Health Statistics, Centers for Disease Control and Prevention, accessed October 30, 2019, U.S. Department of Health and Human Services, www.cdc.gov/nchs; Table 1. Deaths, percentage of total deaths, and death rates for the ten leading causes of death in selected age groups, by race and Hispanic origin and sex: United States, 2017, National Vital Statistics Reports, Deaths: Leading Causes for 2017, Volume 68, No. 6, National Center for Health Statistics, Centers for Disease Control and Prevention, June 24, 2019, U.S. Department of Health and Human Services, www.cdc.gov/nchs.

[14] Deaths and Death Rates for the 10 Leading Causes of Death, by Sex: United States, 1976, National

Center for Health Statistics, accessed August 8, 2019, Centers for Disease Control and Prevention, U.S. Department of Health and Human Services, www.cdc.gov/nchs.

[15] Henry I. Russek, MD and Burton L. Zohman, MD, "Chances for Survival in Acute Myocardial Infarction," Journal of the American Medical Association, October 23, 1954, American Medical Association, www.jamanetwork.com; A. Maziar Zafari, MD et al, "What is the prognosis of acute myocardial infarction (MI, heart attack)?," Medscape, May 7, 2019, www.emedicine.medscape.com.

[16] Deaths and Death Rates for the 10 Leading Causes of Death, by Sex: United States, 1976, National Center for Health Statistics, accessed August 8, 2019, Centers for Disease Control and Prevention, U.S. Department of Health and Human Services, www.cdc.gov/nchs; 10 Leading Causes of Death, United States / 2019 / All Races, Both Sexes, National Center for Injury Prevention and Control, National Center for Health Statistics, Centers for Disease Control and Prevention, February 20, 2020, U.S. Department of Health and Human Services, www.cdc.gov/nchs; Stacy Simon, "Facts & Figures 2019: U.S. Cancer Death Rate Has Dropped 27% in 25 Years," American Cancer Society, January 8, 2019, www.cancer.org; "Heart Disease and Stroke Statistics—2019 Update: A Report from the American Heart Association," American Heart Association Circulation Journal, March 5, 2019, American Heart Association, www.ahajournals.org; "Yesterday, Today & Tomorrow: NIH Research Timelines / Stroke," Research Portfolio Online Reporting Tools, National Institutes of Health, accessed October 15, 2019, U.S. Department of Health and Human Services, www.nih.gov.

[17] Stephanie Bernell and Steven W. Howard, "Use Your Words Carefully: What is a Chronic Disease?," Frontiers in Public Health, August 2, 2016, www.frontiersin.org; "About Chronic Diseases," National Center for Chronic Disease Prevention and Health Promotion (NCCDPHP), Centers for Disease Control and Prevention, January 12, 2021, U.S. Department of Health and Human Services, www.cdc.gov; Jill Ashman, PhD et al, Characteristics of Office-based Physician Visits, 2016, NCHS Data Brief, No. 331, National Center for Health Statistics, Centers for Disease Control and Prevention, January 2019, U.S. Department of Health and Human Services, www.cdc.gov/nchs.

[18] "Health – United States – 1976-1977," Public Health Service, Health Resources Administration, 1977, U.S. Department of Health, Education and Welfare, www.cdc.gov; "Chronic Diseases in America," National Center for Chronic Disease Prevention and Health Promotion (NCCDPHP), Centers for Disease Control and Prevention, September 24, 2020, U.S. Department of Health and Human Services, www.cdc.gov; Christine Buttorff, Multiple Chronic Conditions in the United States, Chapter 1 / Prevalence of Multiple Chronic Conditions, Rand Corporation, 2017, www.rand.org; "One of Four Americans Have Multiple Chronic Conditions," Medical Expenditure Panel Survey, Johns Hopkins University Partnership for Solutions, Johns Hopkins University and Robert Wood Johnson Foundation, 2001, www.partnershipforsolutions.org.

[19] "Promoting Health for Children and Adolescents," National Center for Chronic Disease Prevention and Health Promotion, Centers for Disease Control and Prevention (NCCDPHP), accessed October 1, 2020, U.S. Department of Health and Human Services, www.cdc.gov.

[20] "Chronic Kidney Disease in the United States, 2019," Centers for Disease Control and Prevention, March 5, 2019, U.S. Department of Health and Human Services, www.cdc.gov; "Kidney Disease: The Basics," National Kidney Foundation, 2019, www.kidney.org.

[21] E. J. Benjamin et al, "Heart Disease and Stroke Statistics—2019 Update: A Report from the American Heart Association," Circulation, March 5, 2019, American Heart Association, www.ahajournals.org; Salim S. Virani MD, PhD, FAHA et al, "AHA Statistical Update – Heart Disease and Stroke Statistics – 2021 Update," Circulation, February 23, 2021, American Heart Association, www.ahajournals.org.

[22] "By the Numbers – Heart Failure – Facts and Stats," WebMD Focus on Heart Failure, July/August 2018, WebMD, www.webmd.com.

[23] Salim S. Virani MD, PhD, FAHA et al, "AHA Statistical Update – Heart Disease and Stroke Statistics – 2021 Update," Circulation, February 23, 2021, American Heart Association, www.ahajournals.org; "Yesterday, Today & Tomorrow: NIH Research Timelines / Stroke," Research Portfolio Online Reporting Tools, National Institutes of Health, accessed October 15, 2019, U.S. Department of Health and Human

Services, www.nih.gov.
[24] "Diabetes Statistics," National Institute of Diabetes and Digestive and Kidney Diseases, December 2020, U.S. Department of Health and Human Services, www.niddk.nih.gov.
[25] "Cancer Statistics," National Cancer Institute, September 25, 2020, U.S. Department of Health and Human Services, www.cancer.gov.
[26] "High Cholesterol Facts," Centers for Disease Control and Prevention, September 8, 2020, U.S. Department of Health and Human Services, www.cdc.gov.
[27] "Views on End-of-Life Medical Treatments," Pew Research Center, November 21, 2013, www.pewforum.org.
[28] "Death with Dignity Legislation," FAQs – Physician-Hastened Death, accessed October 23, 2020, Death with Dignity, www.deathwithdignity.org.
[29] "14th Amendment to the U.S. Constitution: Civil Rights (1868)," Primary Documents in American History, Library of Congress. www.loc.gov.
[30] Michelle Wandler, "The History of the Informed Consent Requirement in United States Federal Policy," Harvard Library, April 12, 2001, Harvard University, www.dash.Harvard.edu; Olubukunola Mary Tawose, "The Legal Boundaries of Informed Consent," AMA Journal of Ethics, August 2008, American Medical Association, www.journalofethics.ama-assn.org.
[31] Population Estimates – Estimates of the Population of States, by Age – 1965 to 1967, Bureau of the Census, April 17, 1969, U.S. Department of Commerce, www.census.gov.
[32] James R. Wetzel, "American Families: 75 Years of Change," Monthly Labor Review, March 1990; AVG1. Average Number of People per Household, by Race and Hispanic Origin, Marital Status, Age, and Education of Householder, 2019, U.S. Census Bureau, November 2019, U.S. Department of Commerce, www.census.gov; Table HH-4. Households by Size, 1960 to present, U.S. Bureau of the Census, November 2019, U.S. Department of Commerce, www.census.gov.
[33] Historical Census of Housing Tables / Living Alone, U.S. Census Bureau, 2000, July 10, 2017, U.S. Department of Commerce, www.census.gov; Renee Stepler, "Led by Baby Boomers, divorce rates climb for America's 50+ population," Pew Research Center, March 9, 2017, www.pewresearch.org; S0103: Population 65 Years and Over in the United States, 2019 American Community Survey, U.S. Census Bureau, 2019, U.S. Department of Commerce, www.census.gov.
[34] Projected 5-Year Age Groups and Sex Composition of the Population, Projections for the United States: 2017-2060, Main Series. Table 3, U.S. Census Bureau, September 2018, U.S. Department of Commerce, www.census.gov.
[35] Table 1-1. Live Births, Birth Rates and Fertility Rates, by Race: United States, 1909-2000, U.S. Census Bureau, August 4, 2003, U.S. Department of Commerce, www.census.gov; Table MS-1. Marital Status of the Population 15 Years Old and Over by Sex, Race and Hispanic Origin: 1950 to Present, U.S. Census Bureau, December 2020, U.S. Department of Commerce, www.census.gov.
[36] Maria T. Carney et al, "Elder Orphans Hiding in Plain Sight: A Growing Vulnerable Population," Current Gerontology and Geriatrics Research, October 2016, www.hindawi.com.
[37] "Default Surrogate Consent Statutes – September 2019," Commission on Law and Aging, September 2019, American Bar Association, www.americanbar.org.

CHAPTER THREE

[38] "Victory! Americans Everywhere Celebrated the End of World War II in 1945," Prologue Magazine, September 2, 2015, National Archives, www.archives.gov; "U.S. Military Personnel (1939-1945)," National World War II Museum, accessed October 29, 2019, www.nationalww2museum.org.
[39] "The Boomer Stats," BBHQ Boomer Essays: Boomer Statistics (statistics from the U.S. Department of Commerce, Bureau of the Census), Baby Boomer HeadQuarters, accessed October 19, 2019, www.bbhq.com.
[40] Resident Population – estimates by age, sex, race: July 1, 1929, U.S. Census Bureau, October 1, 2004, U.S. Department of Commerce, www.census.gov; "Births Underlying Each Generation," PEW Research Center, December 2015, www.assets.pewresearch.org; Sandra L. Colby and Jennifer Ortman, "The Baby

Boom Cohort in the United States: 2012 to 2060," U.S. Census Bureau, May 2014, U.S. Department of Commerce, www.census.gov.
[41] "Hula Hoop," How Products are Made, Volume 6, www.madehow.com.
[42] Table 3. School enrollment and school enrollment rates, by age and sex: 1940 to 1991," 120 Years of American Education: A Statistical Portrait, Office of Educational Research and Improvement, National Center for Education Statistics, January 1993, U.S. Department of Education, www.ed.gov; Amy F. Ogata, "Building for Learning in Postwar American Elementary Schools," Journal of the Society of Architectural Historians, Volume 67, No. 4, December 2008, Society of Architectural Historians, www.sah.org.
[43] Table 8A. New Single-family and Existing Single-Family Home Prices: 1963-Present and Table 8B. Existing Single-family Home Prices: 1968-Present, U.S. Housing Market Conditions – Historical Data, Office of Policy Development and Research, 1997, Department of Housing and Urban Development and Department of Commerce, www.hud.gov.
[44] Brian Loy, CFA, CFP, "Financial Planning – A Historical Summary and Insights for the Future," Sage Financial Advisors, www.sagefinancialadvisors.com.
[45] "Inductions (by year) from World War I through the end of the draft (1973)," Selective Service System, accessed October 30, 2019, www.sss.gov.
[46] "Draft age is lowered to 18," This Day in History, November 11, The History Channel, November 5, 2009, www.history.com.
[47] "Vietnam Conflict Extract Data File," National Archives, January 2018, www.archives.gov; Combat Area Casualty File, Center for Electronic Records, National Archives, U.S. National Archives and Records Administration, November 1993, www.archives.gov; Vietnam War Deaths, Casualties by Age – Enlisted, American War Library, accessed February 19, 2021, www.americanwarlibrary.com.
[48] Historical Highlights – The 26th Amendment, U.S. House of Representatives: History, Art & Archives, July 1, 1971, U.S. House of Representatives, www.house.gov; "Passage, Ratification and Effects of the 26th Amendment," The History Channel, accessed October 24, 2019, www.history.com.
[49] Projected Age Groups and Sex Composition of the Population, Projections for the United States 2017-2060, Main Series. Table 2, and Projected 5-Year Age Groups and Sex Composition of the Population, Projections for the United States 2017-2060, Main Series. Table 3, U.S. Census Bureau, March 2018, U.S. Department of Commerce, www.census.gov.
[50] Jonathan Vespa et al, "Demographic Turning Points for the United States: Population Projections for 2020 to 2060 / Population Estimates and Projections," Current Population Reports, U.S. Census Bureau, February 2020, U.S. Department of Commerce, www.census.gov.
[51] "Sixty-five Plus in the United States," Economics and Statistics Administration, U.S. Census Bureau, May 1995, U.S. Department of Commerce, www.selectusa.gov.
[52] 2020 Profile of Older Americans, Administration for Community Living, Administration on Aging, May 2020, U.S. Department of Health and Human Services, www.acl.gov.
[53] "2020 Alzheimer's Disease Facts and Figures," Alzheimer's & Dementia, Journal of the Alzheimer's Association, March 2020, Alzheimer's Association, www.alz.org.
[54] Table 15. Functional limitation among adults aged 18 and over, by selected characteristics: United States, selected years 2010-2017, Health, United States – 2018, Centers for Disease Control and Prevention, October 30, 2019, U.S. Department of Health and Human Services, www.cdc.gov.
[55] "Cardiovascular diseases affect nearly half of American adults, statistics show," American Heart Association News, January 31, 2019, American Heart Association, www.heart.org.
[56] Cheryl D. Fryar, MSPH et al, "Prevalence of Overweight, Obesity, and Severe Obesity Among Adults Aged 20 and Over: United States, 1960-1962 Through 2015-2016," Health E-Stats, National Center for Health Statistics, Centers for Disease Control and Prevention, September 2018, U.S. Department of Health and Human Services, www.cdc.gov; Zachary J. Ward, MPH et al, "Projected U.S. State-Level Prevalence of Adult Obesity and Severe Obesity," The New England Journal of Medicine, December 19, 2019, Massachusetts Medical Society,www.nejm.org.
[57] The Health of America / The Health of Millennials, April 24, 2019, Blue Cross/Blue Shield,

www.bcbs.com; The Economic Consequences of Millennial Health, BlueCross/BlueShield / The Health of America, prepared by Moody's Analytics, November 6, 2019, www.bcbs.com.

[58] "Millennials and healthcare: 25 things to know," Becker's Hospital Review, August 4, 2015, www.beckershospitalreview.com; David M. Levine, MD, MPH, MA et al, "Characteristics of Americans With Primary Care and Changes Over Time, 2002-2015," Journal of Internal Medicine, March 2020, American Medical Association, www.jamanetwork.com.

[59] John Virostko, PhD et al, "Recent Trends in the Age of Diagnosis of Colorectal Cancer in the US National Cancer Data Base, 2004-2015," Cancer, March 2019, American Cancer Society, www.cancer.org; "Colorectal Cancer Facts & Figures 2020-2022, American Cancer Society, March 2020, www.cancer.org.

[60] Kathleen Goss, PhD, "New guidelines lower colorectal screening age from 50 to 45," University of Chicago Medicine, May 13, 2018, www.uchicagomedicine.org; American Cancer Society Guideline for Colorectal Cancer Screening, American Cancer Society, November 17, 2020, www.cancer.org; "Why is Colorectal Cancer Rising Rapidly among Young Adults?," National Cancer Institute, November 5, 2020, U.S. Department of Health and Human Services, www. cancer.gov.

[61] James Perrin, MD et al, "The Increase of Childhood Chronic Conditions in the United States," Journal of the American Medical Association, June 27, 2017, American Medical Association, www.jamanetwork.com; America's Children in Brief: Key National Indicators of Well-Being, 2020 – Americas Children at a Glance, Forum on Child and Family Statistics, Federal Interagency Forum on Child and Family Statistics, September 23, 2020, www.childstats.gov; "Promoting Health for Children and Adolescents," National Center for Chronic Disease Prevention and Health Promotion (NCCDPHP), Centers for Disease Control and Prevention, October 1, 2020, U.S. Department of Health and Human Services, www.cdc.gov.

[62] Linda J. Andes, PhD et al, "Prevalence of Prediabetes Among Adolescents and Young Adults in the United States, 2005-2016," Journal of the American Medical Association, December 2, 2019, American Medical Association, www.jamanetwork.com.

[63] Crescent B. Martin, MPH, MA et al, "Prescription Drug Use in the United States, 2015-2016," National Center for Health Statistics, Centers for Disease Control and Prevention, May 2019, U.S. Department of Health and Human Services, www.cdc.gov.

[64] Table 18. Presence of selected chronic conditions at office visits, by patient age and sex: United States, 2016, National Ambulatory Medical Care Survey: 2016 National Summary Tables, National Center for Health Statistics, Centers for Disease Control and Prevention, 2016, U.S. Department of Health and Human Services, www.cdc.gov.

[65] Christine Buttorff et al, Multiple Chronic Conditions in the United States, Rand Corporation, 2017, www.rand.org; "About Chronic Diseases," National Center for Chronic Disease Prevention and Health Promotion (NCCDPHP), Centers for Disease Control and Prevention, accessed October 7, 2020, U.S. Department of Health and Human Services, www.cdc.gov; "One in Four Americans Have Multiple Chronic Conditions," Chronic Conditions: Making the Case for Ongoing Care, Johns Hopkins University Partnership for Solutions, Johns Hopkins University and Robert Wood Johnson Foundation, 2001, www.partnershipforsolutions.org; Brian W. Ward, PhD and Jeannine S. Schiller, MPH, "Prevalence of Multiple Chronic Conditions Among US Adults: Estimates From the National Health Interview Survey, 2010," Preventing Chronic Disease, Centers for Disease Control and Prevention, April 25, 2013, accessed November 6, 2019, U.S. Department of Health and Human Services, www.cdc.gov.

[66] Table 1. Deaths, percentage of total deaths, and death rates for the 10 leading causes of death in selected age groups, by race and Hispanic origin and sex: United States, 2017, National Vital Statistics Reports, Vol. 68, No 6, Centers for Disease Control and Prevention, June 24, 2019, U.S. Department of Health and Human Services, www.cdc.gov; Table 1. Deaths, percentage of total deaths, and death rates for the 10 leading causes of death in selected age groups, by race and sex: United States, 2000, National Vital Statistics Reports, Vol. 50, No 16, Centers for Disease Control and Prevention, September 16, 2002, U.S. Department of Health and Human Services, www.cdc.gov.

[67] Elizabeth Burns, MPH and Ramakrishna Kakara, MPH, "Deaths from Falls Among Persons Aged >65 Years – United States, 2007-2016," Morbidity and Mortality Weekly Report (MMWR), Centers for Disease Control and Prevention, May 11, 2018, U.S. Department of Heath and Human Services, www.cdc.gov; 2019, United States / Unintentional Injuries / Ages 65-85+, All Races, Both Sexes, National Center for Injury Prevention and Control, National Center for Health Statistics, Centers for Disease Control and Prevention, February 20, 2020, U.S. Department of Health and Human Services, www.census.gov; Klaas A. Hartholt, MD, PhD et al, "Mortality From Falls Among U.S. Adults Aged 75 Years or Older, 2000-2016," Journal of the American Medical Association, July 4, 2019, American Medical Association, www.jamanetwork.org.
[68] Briana Moreland, MPH et al, "Trends in Nonfatal Falls and Fall-related Injuries Among Adults Aged 65 and Older – United States 2012-2018," Morbidity and Mortality Weekly Report (MMWR), Centers for Disease Control and Prevention, July 10, 2020, U.S. Department of Health and Human Services, www.cdc.gov; "Take a Stand on Falls," National Center for Injury Prevention & Control, Centers for Disease Control and Prevention, September 22, 2017, U.S. Department of Health and Human Services, www.cdc.gov; "Hip Fractures Among Older Adults," Home and Recreational Safety, Centers for Disease Control and Prevention, accessed October 26, 2020, U.S. Department of Health and Human Services, www.cdc.gov.
[69] "Millennials Outnumber Baby Boomers and Are Far More Diverse, Census Bureau Reports," U.S. Census Bureau Press Release, U.S. Census Bureau, June 25, 2015, U.S. Department of Commerce, www.census.gov.
[70] Projected Population Size and births, Deaths, and Migration, Projections for the United States, 2017-2060, Main Series, Table 1, U.S. Census Bureau, September 2018, U.S. Department of Commerce, www.census.gov.
[71] Christine Eibner et al, "Current and Projected Characteristics and Unique Health Care Needs of the Patient Population Served by the Department of Veterans Affairs," Rand Health Quarterly, Volume 5, No. 4, May 9, 2016, Rand Corporation, www.rand.org; Maria Olenick et al, "U.S. veterans and their unique issues: enhancing health care professional awareness," Advances in Medical Education and Practice, Volume 6, December 2015, www.dovepress.com; "Presumptive Disability Benefits," Veterans Benefits Administration, November 2018, U.S. Department of Veterans Affairs, www.va.gov.
[72] "Veterans' Diseases Associated with Agent Orange," Public Health, accessed December 7, 2019, U.S. Department of Veterans Affairs, www.va.gov; Committee to Review the Health Effects in Vietnam Veterans of Exposure to Herbicides (Eleventh Biennial Update), Veterans and Agent Orange / Update 11 (2018), The National Academies Press, 2018, National Academies of Sciences, Engineering, and Medicine, www.nap.edu.
[73] Raymond Chung, MD, "Baby boomers and hepatitis C: What's the connection?" Harvard Health Publishing, May 1, 2019, Harvard Medical School, www.health.harvard.edu; "Screening Veterans for Hepatitis C Infection," Viral Hepatitis and Liver Disease, accessed November 11, 2019, U.S. Department of Veterans Affairs, www.va.gov.
[74] Service-connected Disability – Rating Status and Ratings for Civilian Veterans 18 Years and Over, U.S. Census Bureau, 2019 American Community Survey 1-year Estimates, U.S. Census Bureau, October 20, 2020, U.S. Department of Commerce, www.census.gov.
[75] 2019 National Veteran Suicide Prevention Annual Report, Office of Mental Health and Suicide Prevention, 2019, U.S. Department of Veterans Affairs, www.va.gov.
[76] Christine Eibner at al, "Current and Projected Characteristics and Unique Health Care Needs of the Patient Population Service by the Department of Veterans Affairs," RAND Health, sponsored by the U.S. Department of Veterans Affairs, 2016, Rand Corporation, www.rand.org; Veteran Population, National Center for Veterans Analysis and Statistics, Congressional Briefing, May 3, 2019, U.S. Department of Veterans Affairs, www.va.gov.
[77] Committee to Review the Health Effects in Vietnam Veterans of Exposure to Herbicides (Eleventh Biennial Update), Veterans and Agent Orange / Update 11 (2018), The National Academies Press, 2018,

National Academies of Sciences, Engineering, and Medicine, www.nap.edu; Coleen A. Boyle et al, Postservice Mortality Among Vietnam Veterans, Centers for Disease Control and Prevention, February 1987, U.S. Department of Health and Human Services, www.cdc.gov; Tegan K. Catlin Boehmer et al, "Postservice mortality in Vietnam veterans: 30-year follow-up," JAMA Internal Medicine, September 27, 2004, American Medical Association, www.jamanetwork.com.

[78] Table 1L: VETPOP2018 Living Veterans by Age Group, Gender, 2018-2048, Predictive Analytics Service, Office of Enterprise Integration, May 2020, U.S. Department of Veterans Affairs, www.va.gov; Erin Bagalman, "The Number of Veterans That Use VA Health Care Services: A Fact Sheet," Congressional Research Service, June 3, 2014, www.crs.gov; Z. Joan Wang, PhD et al, Table 2-2. Enrollees by age group, 2019 Survey of Veteran Enrollees' Health and Use of Health Care – Data Findings Report, VHA Office of Policy and Planning, Veterans Health Administration, March 2020, U.S. Department of Veterans Affairs, www.va.gov; Jonathan E. Vespa, "Those Who Served: America's Veterans From World War II to the War On Terror," U.S. Census Bureau, June 2020, U.S. Department of Commerce, www.census.gov.

CHAPTER FOUR

[79] Sandra L. Colby and Jennifer Ortman, "The Baby Boom Cohort in the United States: 2012 to 2060 / Population Estimates and Projections," U.S. Census Bureau, May 2014, U.S. Department of Commerce, www.census.gov.

[80] Jennifer M. Ortman and Victoria A. Velkoff, "An Aging Nation: The Older Population in the United States / Population Estimates and Projections," U.S. Census Bureau, May 2014, U.S. Department of Commerce, www.census.gov.

[81] "Older People Projected to Outnumber Children for First Time in U.S. History," Release Number CB18-41, U.S. Census Bureau, March 13, 2018, U.S. Department of Commerce, www.census.gov.

[82] Occupational Outlook Handbook: U.S. Bureau of Labor Statistics, April 17, 2020, U.S. Department of Labor, www.bls.gov; Occupational Employment Statistics, Bureau of Labor Statistics, April 17, 2020, U.S. Department of Labor, www.bls.gov.

[83] "Careers in Medicine," The Association of American Medical Colleges, 2019, www.aamc.org.

[84] Aaron Young, PhD et al, "FSMB Census of Licensed Physicians in the United States, 2018," Journal of Medical Regulation, July 2019, Federal of State Medical Boards, www.fsmb.org; 2019 State Physician Workforce Data Report, Association of American Medical Colleges, November 2019, www.aamc.org; The State of Primary Care in the United States / A Chartbook of Facts and Statistics, Robert Graham Center, Policy Studies in Family Medicine and Primary Care, January 2018, www.robert-graham.org; Occupational Outlook Handbook, Bureau of Labor Statistics, September 1, 2020, U.S. Department of Labor, www.bls.gov.

[85] "Professionally Active Primary Care Physicians by Field," The Henry J. Kaiser Family Foundation, March 2019, www.kff.org; Addressing the Nation's Primary Care Shortage: Addressing the Nation's Primary Care Shortage: Advanced Practice Clinicians and Innovative Care Delivery Models, UnitedHealth Group, September 2018, www.unitedhealthgroup.com.

[86] 2018 National Sample Survey of Registered Nurses, Health Resources and Services Administration, National Center for Health Workforce Analysis, January 2020, U.S. Department of Health and Human Services, www.bhw.hrsa.gov; Number of Active RN Licenses by State, National Council of State Boards of Nursing, 2019, www.ncsbn.org; The 2017 National Nursing Workforce Survey, Journal of Nursing Regulation, October 2018, www.journalofnursingregulation.com; Occupational Outlook Handbook, Bureau of Labor Statistics, September 1, 2020, U.S. Department of Labor, www.bls.gov.

[87] Kezia Scales, PhD, "It's Time to Care: A Detailed Profile of America's Direct Care Workforce," PHI (fka National Paraprofessional Healthcare Institute), January 2020, www.phinational.org; Occupational Employment Statistics, Bureau of Labor Statistics, April 17, 2020, U.S. Department of Labor, www.bls.gov; Occupational Outlook Handbook: U.S. Bureau of Labor Statistics, April 17, 2020, U.S. Department of Labor, www.bls.gov.

[88] Occupational Outlook Handbook: Healthcare Occupations, U.S. Bureau of Labor Statistics, April 9,

2021, U.S. Department of Labor, www.bls.gov.
[89] 2019 Review of Physician and Advanced Practitioner Recruiting Incentives, Merritt Hawkins, an AMN Healthcare Company, July 8, 2019, www.merritthawkins.com; Stephen Campbell et al, "Caring for the Future: The Power and Potential of America's Direct Care Workforce," PHI (formerly Paraprofessional Healthcare Institute), January 12, 2020, www.phinational.org.
[90] "Insights from Monthly Employment Data through October 2019," Health Sector Economic Indicators, November 15, 2019, Altarum Center for Value in Health Care, www.altarum.org.
[91] "Insights from Monthly Employment Data through September 2020," Health Sector Economic Indicators, October 16, 2020, Altarum Center for Value in Health Care, www.altarum.org.
[92] Earlene K. P. Dowell, "Census Bureau's 2018 County Business Patterns Providers Data on Over 1,200 Industries," U.S. Census Bureau, October 14, 2020, U.S. Department of Commerce, www.census.gov.
[93] Job openings, hires, and quits reach historic highs in 2019, Monthly Labor Review, U.S. Bureau of Labor Statistics, June 2020, U.S. Department of Labor, www.bls.gov.
[94] 2019 National Health Care Retention & RN Staffing Report, NSI Nursing Solutions, Inc., 2019, www.nsinursingsolutions.com; Ashvin Gandhi et al, "High Nursing Staff Turnover In Nursing Homes Offers Important Quality Information," Health Affairs, March 11, 2021, Project HOPE, The People-to-People Health Foundation, Inc., www.healthaffairs.org.
[95] Staffing and Vacancy Reporting under the MISSION Act of 2018, Department of Veterans Affairs, Office of Inspector General, VA OIG 19-00266-141, June 25, 2019, Department of Veterans Affairs, www.va.gov; "VA releases data on vacancies as required under MISSION Act," Office of Public Affairs – Media Relations, August 31, 2018, U.S. Department of Veterans Affairs, www.va.gov.
[96] Robert Holly, "Home Care Industry Turnover Reaches All-Time High of 82%," Home Health Care News, May 8, 2019, www.homehealthcarenews.com; Aaron Marcum, "Letter From Aaron Marcum: The 2019 Home Care Benchmarking Study," Home Care Pulse, May 7, 2019, www.homecarepulse.com; Kezia Scales, PhD, "It's Time to Care: A Detailed Profile of America's Direct Care Workforce," PHI, January 2020, www.phinational.org.
[97] "Physician Supply and Demand Fact Sheet," Merritt Hawkins White Paper Series, October 31, 2018, Merritt Hawkins, an AMN Healthcare Company, www.merritthawkins.com.
[98] "Primary Medical HPSA Totals," Designated Health professional Shortage Areas Statistics, Second Quarter of Fiscal Year 2021 / Designated HPSA Quarterly Summary, Health Resources and Services Administration (HRSA), March 31, 2021, U.S. Department of Health and Human Services, www.data.hrsa.gov.
[99] "Dental HPSA Totals," Designated Health professional Shortage Areas Statistics, Second Quarter of Fiscal Year 2021 / Designated HPSA Quarterly Summary, Health Resources and Services Administration (HRSA), March 31, 2021, U.S. Department of Health and Human Services, www.data.hrsa.gov; "Mental Health HPSA Totals," Designated Health professional Shortage Areas Statistics, Second Quarter of Fiscal Year 2021 / Designated HPSA Quarterly Summary, Health Resources and Services Administration (HRSA), March 31, 2021, U.S. Department of Health and Human Services, www.data.hrsa.gov.
[100] Mark Murray, MD et al, "Panel Size: How Many Patients Can One Doctor Manage?" Family Practice Management, April 2007, American Academy of Family Physicians, www.aafp.org.
[101] David Ollier Weber, "How Many Patients Can a Primary Care Physician Treat?" American Association for Physician Leadership, February 11, 2019, www.physicianleaders.org; Melanie Raffoul et al, "A Primary Care Panel Size of 2500 is Neither Accurate nor Reasonable," Journal of the American Board of Family Medicine, July 2016, American Board of Family Medicine, www.jabfm.org; Justin Altschuler, MD et al, "Estimating a Reasonable Patient Panel Size for Primary Care Physicians With Team-Based Task Delegation," Annals of Family Medicine, September/October 2012, American Academy of Family Physicians et al, www.annfammed.org.
[102] Brian G. Arndt, MD et al, "Tethered to the EHR: Primary Care Physician Work-load Assessment Using EHR Event Log Data and Time-Motion Observations," Annals of Family Medicine, September/October 2017, American Academy of Family Physicians et al, www.annfammed.org; Richard A. Young, MD et

al, "A Time-Motion Study of Primary Care Physicians' Work in the Electronic Health Record Era," Family Medicine, February 2018, Society of Teachers of Family Medicine, www.journals.stfm.org; Linda W. Higgins, PhD, RN et al, "Hospital Nurses' Work Activity in a Technology-Rich Environment," Journal of Nursing Care Quality, November 10, 2016, Clinical Nurse Leader Association, www.cnlassociation.org.

[103] 2018 Survey of America's Physicians, Practice Patterns and Perspectives, conducted by Merritt Hawkins and AMN Healthcare, September 2018, The Physicians Foundation, www.physiciansfoundation.org; 90th Annual Physician Report: Despite challenges, doctors remain productive, Medical Economics, April 17, 2019, www.medicaleconomics.com.

[104] 2017 Survey of Physician Appointment Wait Times and Medicare and Medicaid Acceptance Rates, Merritt Hawkins, August 31, 2017, Merritt Hawkins, an AMN Health Care Company, www.merritthawkins.com.

[105] Dale Lupu, MPH, PhD et al, "The Growing Demand for Hospice and Palliative Medicine Physicians: Will the Supply Keep Up?" Journal of Pain Symptom Management, April 2018, American Academy of Hospice and Palliative Medicine, www.aahpm.org.

[106] Jill J. Ashman, PhD et al, "Characteristics of Office-based Physician Visits, 2016," National Center for Health Statistics, January 2019, Centers for Disease Control and Prevention, U.S. Department of Health and Human Services, www.cdc.gov/nchs.

[107] Amy Symens Smith and Edward Trevelyan, "The Older Population in Rural America: 2012-2016 – American Community Survey Reports" U.S. Census Bureau, September 2019, U.S. Department of Commerce, www.census.gov.

[108] Table 18, Presence of selected chronic conditions at office visits, by patient age and sex: United States, 2016, National Ambulatory Medical Care Survey: 2016 National Summary Tables, accessed October 18, 2019, National Center for Health Statistics, Centers for Disease Control and Prevention, U.S. Department of Health and Human Services, www.cdc.gov; Arif H. Kamal et al, "Policy Changes Key to Promoting Sustainability and Growth of the Specialty Palliative Care Workforce," Health Affairs, June 2019, Project HOPE, The People-to-People Health Foundation, Inc., www.healthaffairs.org.

[109] Table 1. Projected Population Size and Births, Deaths and Migration, Projections for the United States: 2017 – 2060, U.S. Census Bureau, September 2018, U.S. Department of Commerce, www.census.gov.

[110] "Projections overview and highlights, 2019-29," Monthly Labor Review, September 2020, U.S. Bureau of Labor Statistics, U.S. Department of Labor, www.bls.gov.

[111] Table 1.3 Fast growing occupations, 2019 and projected 2029, "Employment Projections: Fastest growing occupations," U.S. Bureau of Labor Statistics, September 1, 2020, U.S. Department of Labor, www.bls.gov; Employment Projections – 2019-2029, News Release, Occupational Outlook Handbook, Bureau of Labor Statistics, September 1, 2020, U.S. Department of Labor, www.bls.gov.

[112] Handbook of Methods, Employment Projections, accessed September 4, 2019, U.S. Bureau of Labor Statistics, U.S. Department of Labor, www.bls.gov; numerous emails and phone conversations between the author and Bureau of Labor Statistics staff in December 2019.

[113] Kezia Scales, PhD, "It's Time to Care: A Detailed Profile of America's Direct Care Workforce," PHI (fka National Paraprofessional Healthcare Institute), January 2020, www.phinational.org.

[114] Occupational Outlook Handbook: Healthcare Occupations, U.S. Bureau of Labor Statistics, April 9, 2021, U.S. Department of Labor, www.bls.gov.

[115] Table 2. Projected Age Groups and Sex Composition of the Population, Projections for the United States 2017-2060, U.S. Census Bureau, March 2018, U.S. Department of Commerce, www.census.gov.

[116] Stephen Campbell et al, "Caring for the Future: The Power and Potential of America's Direct Care Workforce," PHI (formerly Paraprofessional Healthcare Institute), January 21, 2020, www.phinational.org.

[117] Ruirui Sun, PhD et al, "Trends in Hospital Emergency Department Visits by Age and Payer, 2006-2015," Healthcare Cost and Utilization Project (HCUP), Agency for Healthcare Research and Quality, March 2018, U.S. Department of Health and Human Services, www.hcup-us.ahrq.gov.

[118] Jill J. Ashman, PhD et al, "Characteristics of Office-based Physician Visits, 2016," National Center for

Health Statistics, January 2019, Centers for Disease Control and Prevention, U.S. Department of Health and Human Services, www.cdc.gov/nchs.
[119] 2019 Update – The Complexities of Physician Supply and Demand: Projections from 2017 to 2032, submitted by HIS Markit Ltd., April 2019, Association of American Medical Colleges, www.aamc.org; .
[120] 2019 State Physician Workforce Data Report, November 2019, Association of American Medical Colleges, www.aamc.org; Arif H. Kamal, MD, MBA, MHS et al, "Future of the Palliative Care Workforce: Preview to an Impending Crisis," The American Journal of Medicine, February 2017, Alliance for Academic Internal Medicine, www.amjmed.com; 2019 Update – The Complexities of Physician Supply and Demand: Projections from 2017 to 2032, submitted by HIS Markit Ltd., April 2019, Association of American Medical Colleges, www.aamc.org; The Future of Healthcare – A National Survey of Physicians - 2018, The Doctors Company, Medical Malpractice Insurance, 2018, www.thedoctors.com.
[121] Table 15. Employed persons by detailed occupation, sex, and age, Annual Average 2018 (Source: Current Population Survey), U.S. Bureau of Labor Statistics, January 2019. U.S. Department of Labor, www.bls.gov; Aaron Young, PhD et al, "FSMB Census of Licensed Physicians in the United States, 2018," Journal of Medical Regulation, July 2019, Federal of State Medical Boards, www.fsmb.org; Arif H. Kamal, MD, MBA, MHS et al, "Policy Changes Key to Promoting Sustainability and Growth of the Specialty Palliative Care Workforce," Health Affairs, June 2019, Project HOPE, The People-to-People Health Foundation, Inc., www.healthaffairs.org; Table 2: Demographic Characteristics of AAFP Members, American Association of Family Practitioners, December 2018, www.aafp.org; White Paper Series, The Aging Physician Workforce, 2018, Merritt Hawkins, an AMN Healthcare Company, www.merritthawkins.com; Growing Shortage of Rheumatologists "Very Concerning" – News, Arthritis Foundation, February 20, 2020, www.arthritis.org.
[122] 2018 National Sample Survey of Registered Nurses, Bureau of Health Workforce, National Center for Health Workforce Analysis, January 2020, Health Resources and Services Administration, U.S. Department of Health and Human Services, www.bhw.hrsa.gov; Richard A Smiley, MS MA et al, The 2017 National Nursing Workforce Survey, Journal of Nursing Regulation, October 2018, National Council of State Boards of Nursing, www.ncsbn.org; The U.S. Nursing Workforce: Trends in Supply and Education," Bureau of Health Professions, National Center for Health Workforce Analysis, October 2013, Health Resources and Services Administration, U.S. Department of Health and Human Services, www.bhw.hrsa.gov.
[123] Peter I. Buerhaus, PhD, RN, FFAN, FANNP et al, "Four Challenges Facing the Nursing Workforce in the United States," Journal of Nursing Regulation, July 2017, National Council of State Boards of Nursing, www.ncsbn.org.
[124] Stephen Campbell et al, "Caring for the Future: The Power and Potential of America's Direct Care Workforce," PHI (formerly Paraprofessional Healthcare Institute), January 21, 2020, www.phinational.org.
[125] Total Number of Medical School Graduates, 2002-2018, Association of American Medical Colleges, 2018, www.aamc.org; 2019 State Physician Workforce Data Report, Association of American Medical Colleges, November 2019, www.aamc.org; Barbara Barzansky, PhD and Sylvia I. Etzel, "Medical Schools in the United States, 2018-2019, Journal of the American Medical Association, September 10, 2019, American Medical Association, www.jamanetwork.com.
[126] Aaron Young, PhD et al, "FSMB Census of Licensed Physicians in the United States, 2018," Journal of Medical Regulation, July 2019, Federal of State Medical Boards, www.fsmb.org.
[127] 2018 Number of Candidates Taking NCLEX Examination and Percent Passing, by Type of Candidate, National Council of State Boards of Nursing, accessed December 19, 2019, www.ncsbn.org; "Number of RN-to-BSN program graduates annually," Campaign for Action, July 9, 2019, www.campaignforaction.org.
[128] 2018-2019 Enrollment and Graduations in Baccalaureate and Graduate Programs in Nursing, American Association of Colleges of Nursing, 2019, www.aacnnursing.org.

[129] National Projections of Supply and Demand for Selected Behavioral Health Practitioners: 2013 – 2025, Health Resources and Service Administration, Bureau of Health Workforce, National Center for Health Workforce Analysis, November 2016, U.S. Department of Health and Human Services, www.hrsa.gov.
[130] The Complexities of Physician Supply and Demand, Projections from 2013 to 2025, Association of American Colleges, March 2015, www.aamc.org.
[131] 2016 Update – The Complexities of Physician Supply and Demand: Projections from 2014 to 2025 – Final Report, Association of American Medical Colleges, April 5, 2016, www.aamc.org.
[132] 2017 Update – The Complexities of Physician Supply and Demand: Projections from 2015 to 2030 – Final Report, Association of American Medical Colleges, February 28, 2017, www.aamc.org.
[133] 2018 Update – The Complexities of Physician Supply and Demand: Projections from 2016 to 2030 – Final Report, Association of American Medical Colleges, March 2018, www.aamc.org.
[134] Matthew Stevenson, "Demand for Healthcare Workers will Outpace Supply by 2025: An Analysis of the U.S. Healthcare Labor Market," Mercer HPA, 2018, Marsh & McLennan Companies, www.mmc.com.
[135] 2019 Update – The Complexities of Physician Supply and Demand: Projections from 2017 to 2032, Association of American Medical Colleges, April 2019, www.aamc.org.
[136] Xiaoming Zhang et al, "Physician workforce in the United States of America: forecasting nationwide shortages," Human Resources for Health, February 6, 2020, BMC/Springer Nature, www.human-resources-health.biomedcentral.com.
[137] The Complexities of Physician Supply and Demand: Projections From 2018 to 2033, Association of American Medical Colleges, June 202, www.aamc.org; The Complexities of Physician Supply and Demand: Projections From 2019 to 2034, Association of American Medical Colleges, June 2021, www.aamc.org.
[138] Stephen P. Juraschek et al, "United States Registered Nurse Workforce Report Card and Shortage Forecast," American Journal of Medical Quality, May/June 2012, American College of Medical Quality, www.acmq.org.
[139] Xiaoming Zhang, PhD et al, "United States Registered Nurse Workforce Report Card and Shortage Forecast: A Revisit," American Journal of Medical Quality, May/June 2018, American College of Medical Quality, www.acmq.org.
[140] National and State-Level Projections of Dentists and Dental Hygienists in the U.S., 2012-2015, Bureau of Health Workforce, National Center for Workforce Analysis, Health Resources and Services Administration, February 2015, U.S. Department of Health and Human Services, www.hrsa.gov.
[141] Vernon W. Lin et al, "U.S. Social Worker Workforce Report Card: Forecasting Nationwide Shortages," Social Work, January 2016, National Association of Social Workers, www.socialworkers.org.
[142] National and Regional Projections of Supply and Demand for Primary Care Practitioners: 2013-2025, Bureau of Health Workforce, National Center for Workforce Analysis, Health Resources and Services Administration, November 2016, U.S. Department of Health and Human Services, www.hrsa.gov.
[143] National Projections of Supply and Demand for Selected Behavioral Health Practitioners: 2013-2025, Bureau of Health Workforce, National Center for Workforce Analysis, Health Resources and Services Administration, November 2016, U.S. Department of Health and Human Services, www.hrsa.gov.
[144] National and Regional Projections of Supply and Demand for Geriatricians: 2013-2025, Bureau of Health Workforce, National Center for Workforce Analysis, Health Resources and Services Administration, April 2017, U.S. Department of Health and Human Services, www.hrsa.gov.
[145] Matthew Stevenson, "Demand for Healthcare Workers Will Outpace Supply by 2025: An Analysis of the U.S. Healthcare Labor Market," Mercer HPA, 2018, Marsh & McLennan Companies, www.mcc.com.
[146] Dale Lupu, et al, "The Growing Demand for Hospice and Palliative Medicine Physicians: Will the Supply Keep Up?" Journal of Pain Symptom Management, April 2018, American Academy of Hospice and Palliative Medicine, www.aahpm.org.
[147] Behavioral Health Workforce Projections, 2016-2030: Psychiatrists (Adult), Child and Adolescent Psychiatrists, Bureau of Health Workforce, National Center for Workforce Analysis, Health Resources and Services Administration, 2019, U.S. Department of Health and Human Services, www.hrsa.gov.

[148] 2019 Update – The Complexities of Physician Supply and Demand: Projections from 2017 to 2032, Association of American Medical Colleges, April 2019, www.aamc.org; The Complexities of Physician Supply and Demand: Projections From 2018 to 2033, Association of American Medical Colleges, June 2020, www.aamc.org; The Complexities of Physician Supply and Demand: Projections From 2019 to 2034, Association of American Medical Colleges, June 2021, www.aamc.org.
[149] Behavioral Health Workforce Projections, 2017-2030: [sic], Bureau of Health Workforce, National Center for Workforce Analysis, Health Resources and Services Administration, 2020, U.S. Department of Health and Human Services, www.hrsa.gov.
[150] The Future of the Nursing Workforce: National- and State-Level Projections, 2012-2025, Bureau of Health Workforce, National Center for Workforce Analysis, Health Resources and Services Administration, April 2017, U.S. Department of Health and Human Services, www.hrsa.gov.
[151] Supply and Demand Projections of the Nursing Workforce: 2014-2030, Bureau of Health Workforce, National Center for Workforce Analysis, Health Resources and Services Administration, July 21, 2017, U.S. Department of Health and Human Services, www.hrsa.gov.
[152] "Allied Health Workforce Projections, 2016-2030: Pharmacists," Bureau of Health Workforce, National Center for Workforce Analysis, Health Resources and Services Administration, 2018, U.S. Department of Health and Human Services, www.hrsa.gov.
[153] "Allied Health Workforce Projections, 2016-2030: Occupational and Physical Therapists," Bureau of Health Workforce, National Center for Workforce Analysis, Health Resources and Services Administration, 2018, U.S. Department of Health and Human Services, www.hrsa.gov.
[154] Behavioral Health Workforce Projections, 2016-2030: Social Workers, Bureau of Health Workforce, National Center for Workforce Analysis, Health Resources and Services Administration, 2019, U.S. Department of Health and Human Services, www.hrsa.gov.
[155] Behavioral Health Workforce Projections, 2016-2030: Psychiatrists (Adult), Child and Adolescent Psychiatrists, Bureau of Health Workforce, National Center for Workforce Analysis, Health Resources and Services Administration, 2019, U.S. Department of Health and Human Services, www.hrsa.gov.
[156] Behavioral Health Workforce Projections, 2017-2030: [sic], Bureau of Health Workforce, National Center for Workforce Analysis, Health Resources and Services Administration, 2020, U.S. Department of Health and Human Services, www.hrsa.gov.
[157] Oral Health Workforce Projections, 2017-2030: Dentists and Dental Hygienists, Bureau of Health Workforce, National Center for Workforce Analysis, Health Resources and Services Administration, 2020, U.S. Department of Health and Human Services, www.hrsa.gov.
[158] Morgan Haefner, "'Overrun with kid attempting suicide': Children's Colorado declares state of emergency," Beckers Hospital Review, May 26, 2021, www.beckershospitalreview.com; State Suicide Rates Among Adolescents and Young Adults Aged 10-24: United States, 2000-2018, National Vital Statistics Reports, Vol. 69, No 11, Centers for Disease Control and Prevention, September 11, 2020, U.S. Department of Health and Human Services, www.cdc.gov.
[159] Designated Health Professional Shortage Areas Statistics, Health Resources and Services Administration, September 30, 2020, U.S. Department of Health and Human Services, www.data.hrsa.gov; Behavioral Health Workforce Projections, 2016-2030: Psychiatrists (Adult), Child and Adolescent Psychiatrists, Bureau of Health Workforce, National Center for Workforce Analysis, Health Resources and Services Administration, 2019, U.S. Department of Health and Human Services, www.hrsa.gov; Technical Documentation for Health Resources Service Administration's Health Workforce Simulation Model, Bureau of Health Workforce, National Center for Workforce Analysis, Health Resources and Services Administration, 2020, U.S. Department of Health and Human Services, www.hrsa.gov.
[160] H. L. Mencken, 1880-1956, American columnist and cultural critic.
[161] National Health Expenditures Fact Sheet, Historical NHE, 2019, U.S. Centers for Medicare and Medicaid Services, December 16, 2020, U.S. Department of Health and Human Services, www.cms.gov; "CMS Office of the Actuary Releases 2018-2027 Projections of National Health Expenditures," U.S.

Centers for Medicare and Medicaid Services (CMS), February 20, 2019, U.S. Department of Health and Human Services, www.cms.gov; "How has U.S. spending on healthcare changed over time?," Peterson-Kaiser Health System Tracker, KFF Analysis of U.S. Department of Health and Human Services Medical Expenditure Panel Survey, December 20, 2019, Peterson Center on Healthcare and Kaiser Family Foundation, www.healthsystemtracker.org.

[162] National Health Expenditures Fact Sheet, Historical NHE, 2019, U.S. Centers for Medicare and Medicaid Services, December 16, 2020, U.S. Department of Health and Human Services, www.cms.gov; Katharine Levit et al, "Inflation Spurs Health Spending in 2000," Health Affairs, January/February 2000, Project HOPE, The People-to-People Health Foundation, Inc., www.healthaffairs.org.

[163] Per person spending – Peterson-Kaiser Health System Tracker, KFF Analysis of U.S. Department of Health and Human Services Medical Expenditure Panel Survey, March 29, 2019, Peterson Center on Healthcare and Kaiser Family Foundation, www.healthsystemtracker.com.

[164] Etienne Gaudette, "Health and Health Care of Medicare Beneficiaries in 2030," Forum for Health Economics and Policy, U.S. National Library of Medicine, National Institutes of Health, April 2016, U.S. Department of Health and Human Services, www.nlm.nih.gov.

[165] Hugh Waters and Marlon Graff, America's Obesity Crisis / The Health and Economic Costs of Excess Weight," Milken Institute, October 2018, 2018, www.milkeninstitute.org; "Chronic Conditions Charts: 2017," U.S. Centers for Medicare and Medicaid Services, 2017, U.S. Department of Health and Human Services, www.cms.gov; Hugh Waters and Marlon Graf, The Costs of Chronic Disease in the U.S., Milken Institute, August 2018, www.milkeninstitute.org; "2020 Alzheimer's Disease Facts and Figures," Alzheimer's & Dementia, Journal of the Alzheimer's Association, March 2020, Alzheimer's Association, www.alz.org.

[166] Medicaid's Role in Nursing Home Care, The Henry J. Kaiser Family Foundation, June 2017, www.kff.org.

[167] "2020 Alzheimer's Disease Facts and Figures," Alzheimer's & Dementia, Journal of the Alzheimer's Association, March 2020, Alzheimer's Association, www.alz.org.

[168] Caregiving in the U.S., AARP and the National Alliance for Caregiving, May 2020, www.AARP.org; Kezia Scales, PhD, "It's Time to Care: A Detailed Profile of America's Direct Care Workforce," PHI (fka National Paraprofessional Healthcare Institute), January 2020, www.phinational.org; "Unpaid Eldercare in the United States – 2017-2018, Data from the American Time Use Survey," U.S. Bureau of Labor Statistics, November 22, 2019, U.S. Department of Labor, www.bls.gov; "2020 Alzheimer's Disease Facts and Figures," Alzheimer's & Dementia, Journal of the Alzheimer's Association, March 2020, Alzheimer's Association, www.alz.org.

[169] "Cost of Older Adult Falls," Centers for Disease Control and Prevention, July 9, 2020, www.cdc.gov; C. S. Florence et al, "Medical Costs of Fatal and Nonfatal Falls in Older Adults, Journal of the American Geriatrics Society, March 2018, American Geriatrics Society, www.americangeriatrics.org.

[170] National Health Expenditures Fact Sheet, Historical NHE, 2019, U.S. Centers for Medicare and Medicaid Services, December 16, 2020, U.S. Department of Health and Human Services, www.cms.gov; A Data Book – Health Care Spending and the Medicare Program, Medicare Advisory Commission (an independent congressional agency authorized under the Balance Budget Act of 1997), July 2020. www.medpac.gov.

[171] Etienne Gaudette, "Health and Health Care of Medicare Beneficiaries in 2030," Forum for Health Economics and Policy, U.S. National Library of Medicine, National Institutes of Health, April 2016, U.S Department of Health and Human Services, www.nlm.nih.gov; National Health Expenditures Fact Sheet, Historical NHE, 2019, U.S. Centers for Medicare and Medicaid Services, December 16, 2020, U.S. Department of Health and Human Services, www.cms.gov.

[172] "How is Medicare funded?" Centers for Medicare and Medicaid Services, accessed January 23, 2020, U.S. Department of Health and Human Services, www.cms.gov; A Data Book – Health Care Spending and the Medicare Program, Medicare Advisory Commission (an independent congressional agency authorized under the Balance Budget Act of 1997), July 2020, www.medpac.gov.

[173] Daria Pelech, An Analysis of Private-Sector Prices for Physicians' Services, Working Paper Series, Congressional Budget Office, January 2018, www.cbo.gov; Chapin White and Christopher Whaley, "Prices Paid to Hospitals by Private Health Plans Are High Relative to Medicare and Vary Widely," Rand Corporation, 2019, www.rand.org.

[174] "Why rural hospitals are closing," Becker's Hospital Review, August 28, 2019, www.beckershospitalreview.com; Ayla Ellison, "State-by-state breakdown of 130 rural hospital closures," Becker's Hospital Review, June 8, 2020, www.beckershospitalreview.com.

[175] Fred Schulte, "Millions of Older Americans Live in Counties With No ICU Beds as Pandemic Intensifies," Kaiser Health News, March 20, 2020, www.khn.org.

[176] Juliette Cubanski et al, "How Much Do Medicare Beneficiaries Spend Out of Pocket on Health Care?," The Henry J. Kaiser Family Foundation, November 4, 2019, www.kff.org; "Understanding Medicare's out-of-pocket costs," Humana, Inc., 2019, www.humana.com; Gretchen Jacobson et al, "A Dozen Facts About Medicare Advantage in 2019," The Henry J. Kaiser Family Foundation, June 6, 2019, www.kff.org.

[177] Juliette Cubanski et al, "Medicare Beneficiaries' Out-of-Pocket Health Care Spending as a Share of Income Now and Projections for the Future," The Henry J. Kaiser Family Foundation, January 26, 2018, www.kff.org.

[178] Bianca DiJulio, "Data Note: Americans' Challenges with Health Care Costs," Kaiser Family Foundation, March 2, 2017, www.kff.org; Renuka Tipirneni, MC, MSc et al, "Health Insurance Affordability Concerns and Health Care Avoidance Among US Adults Approaching Retirement," Journal of the American Medical Association Network Open, February 7, 2020, American Medical Association, www.jamanetwork.com.

[179] National Health Expenditures Fact Sheet, Historical NHE, 2019, U.S. Centers for Medicare and Medicaid Services, December 16, 2020, U.S. Department of Health and Human Services, www.cms.gov; 2018 Health Care Cost and Utilization Report, The Health Care Cost Institute, February 2020, www.healthcostinstitute.org.

[180] "2020 Employer Health Benefits Survey," The Henry J. Kaiser Family Foundation, October 8, 2020, www.kff.org; Matthew Rae et al, "Tracking the rise in premium contributions and cost-sharing for families with large employer coverage," Peterson-KFF Health System Tracker, August 14, 2019, www.healthsystemtracker.com.

CHAPTER FIVE

[181] Paul Kalanithi, When Breath Becomes Air, Random House, New York, 2016, www.penguinrandomhouse.com.

[182] Mark Kutner et al, The Health Literacy of America's Adults – Results from the 2003 National Assessment of Adult Literacy, American Institutes for Research, National Center for Education Statistics, Institute of Education Sciences, September 2006, U.S. Department of Education. www.nces.ed.gov.

[183] Catherine R. Selden, MLS et al, Health Literacy, National Library of Medicine Current Bibliographies in Medicine: Health Literacy, January 1999 through October 1999, U.S. National Library of Medicine, National Institutes of Health, February 2000, U.S Department of Health and Human Services, www.researchgate.net; "Health Literacy Interventions and Outcomes: An Updated Systematic Review," Agency for Healthcare Research and Quality, March 2011, U.S. Department of Health and Human Services, www.ahrq.gov; Philip M. Massey, PhD MPH et al, "Visualizing Patterns and Trends of 25 years of Published Health Literacy Research," Health Literacy Research and Practice, October 2017, Healio, www.healio.com.

[184] The UnitedHealthcare Consumer Sentiment Survey, August 2017, United Healthcare, www.uhc.com.

[185] "Health and Economic Costs of Chronic Diseases," National Center for Chronic Disease Prevention and Health Promotion (NCCDPHP), Centers for Disease Control and Prevention, September 15, 2020, U.S. Department of Health and Human Services, www.cdc.gov.

[186] National Action Plan to Improve Health Literacy, Office of Disease Prevention and Health Promotion, May 2010, U.S. Department of Health and Human Services, www.hhs.gov; Matteo Fabbri, MD et al, "Health Literacy and Outcomes in Patients With Heart Failure: A Prospective Community Study," Mayo

Clinic Proceedings, January 2018, Mayo Clinic, www.mayoclinicproceedings.org; Joseph Boyle, MD et al, "Low Health Literacy is Associated with Increased Transitional Care Needs in Hospitalized Patients," Journal of Hospital Medicine, September 20, 2017, Society of Hospital Medicine, www.journalofhospitalmedicine.com; M. Stellefson et al, "Association Between Health Literacy, Electronic Health Literacy, Disease-specific Knowledge, and Health-Related Quality of Life Among Adults with Chronic Obstructive Pulmonary Disease: Cross-sectional Study," Journal of Medical Internet Research, June 6, 2019, www.jmirpublications.com.

[187] Betty R. Ferrell, PhD, RN, "Live Longer or Better? Cancer Patients Shouldn't Have to Choose," Medscape, July 12, 2018, www.medscape.com; Judith H. Hibbard and Jessica Greene, "What the Evidence Shows About Patient Activation: Better Health Outcomes and Care Experiences: Fewer Data on Costs," Health Affairs, February 2013, Project HOPE, The People-to-People Health Foundation, Inc., www.healthaffairs.org.

[188] "20 Tips to Help Prevent Medical Errors: Patient Fact Sheet," Agency for Healthcare Research and Quality, August 2018, U.S. Department of Health and Human Services, www.ahrq.gov.

[189] R. B. Friedland, "Understanding health literacy: new estimates of the costs of inadequate health literacy", U.S. Government Printing Office, 1998, National Academy on an Aging Society, www.geron.org; Steve Leuck, PharmD, "The Cost of Low Health Literacy," Pharmacy Times, April 10, 2017, www.pharmacytimes.com; Jonathan H. Watanabe, PharmD, MS, PhD et al, "Cost of Prescription Drug-Related Morbidity and Mortality," Annals of Pharmacotherapy, March 26, 2018, www.journals.sagepub.com; The Hidden Cost of Healthcare System Complexity, Accenture, September 2018, www.accenture.com.

CHAPTER SIX

[190] Healthy People, The Surgeon General's Report on Health Promotion and Disease Prevention, U.S. Public Health Service, 1979, U.S. Department of Health, Education and Welfare; Promoting Health / Preventing Disease, Public Health Service, Fall 1980, U.S. Department of Health and Human Services; Promoting Health/Preventing Disease / Objectives for the Nation, National Institute of Education, ducational Resources Information Center (ERIC), Fall 1980, U.S. Department of Education.

[191] Angela K. McGowan et al, "Healthy People: The Role of Law and Policy in the Nation's Public Health Agenda, The Journal of Law, Medicine & Ethics, Summer 2019, American Society of Law, Medicine and Ethics, www.aslme.org.

[192] Healthy People 1990 (published 1980): 226 objectives / 16 percent of objectives met; Healthy People 2000 (published 1990): 376 objectives / 21 percent of objectives met; Healthy People 2010 (published 2000): 969 objectives / 23 percent of objectives met; Healthy People 2020 (published 2010): 1,300 objectives / 26 percent of objectives met. Data from: Healthy People 2000 Final Review, National Center for Health Statistics, October 2001, U.S. Department of Health and Human Services, www.cdc.gov; Healthy People 2010 Final Review, Centers for Disease Control and Prevention, December 2012, U.S. Department of Health and Human Services, www.HealthyPeople.gov; "Healthy People 2020 Final Review," Healthy People 2020: An End of Decade Snapshot [undated], Office of the Assistant Secretary for Health, Office of Disease Prevention and Health Promotion, updated March 16, 2021, accessed June 6, 2021, U.S. Department of Health and Human Services, www.health.gov.

[193] "Progress Reviews for Healthy People 2020," National Center for Health Statistics, Centers for Disease Control and Prevention, U.S. Department of Health and Human Services, accessed February 19, 2020, www.healthypeople.gov; "Healthy People 2020 Final Review," Healthy People 2020: An End of Decade Snapshot [undated], Office of the Assistant Secretary for Health, Office of Disease Prevention and Health Promotion, updated March 16, 2021, accessed June 6, 2021, U.S. Department of Health and Human Services, www.health.gov.

[194] Ending the Tobacco Problem, a Blueprint for the Nation, Committee on Reducing Tobacco Use: Strategies, Barriers, and Consequences, National Academies Press Open Book, 2007, Institute of Medicine of the National Academies, www.nap.edu; "Cigarette smoking is down, but almost 38 million Americans still smoke," Centers for Disease Control and Prevention, January 18, 2018, U.S. Department of Health

and Human Services, www.cdc.gov; Smoking and Tobacco Use, Centers for Disease Control and Prevention, November 16, 2020, U.S. Department of Health and Human Services, www.cdc.gov.

[195] Yang Du, MD, MS et al, "Trends in Adherence to the Physical Activity Guidelines for Americans for Aerobic Activity and Time Spent on Sedentary Behavior Among US Adults, 2007 to 2016," Journal of the American Medical Association, July 26, 2019, American Medical Association, www.jamanetwork.com.

[196] Amy F. Ogata, "Building for Learning in Postwar American Elementary Schools," Journal of the Society of Architectural Historians, Volume 67, No. 4, December 2008, Society of Architectural Historians, www.sah.org.

[197] "History / CMS' [sic] program history," Centers for Medicare and Medicaid Services, accessed January 28, 2020, U.S. Department of Health and Human Services, www.cms.gov.

[198] The Nation's Physician Workforce: Options for Balancing Supply and Requirements, National Academies Press, 1996, Institute of Medicine Committee on the U.S. Physician Supply, Institute of Medicine of the National Academies, www.nap.edu.

[199] Report of the Graduate Medical Education National Advisory Committee to the Secretary, Department of Health and Human Services, Health Resources Administration, September 30, 1980, U.S. Department of Health and Human Services, www.hhs.com.

[200] Physician Payment Review Commission - Annual Report to Congress 1992, Physician Payment Review Commission, 1992 (Physician Payment Review Commission, along with ProPAC, merged into MedPAC in 1998).

[201] The Nation's Physician Workforce: Options for Balancing Supply and Requirements, National Academies Press, Institute of Medicine Committee on the U.S. Physician Supply, 1996, Institute of Medicine of the National Academies, www.nap.edu.

[202] COGME Physician Workforce Policies: Recent Developments and Remaining Challenges in Meeting National Goals, Council on Graduate Medical Education / Fourteenth Report, Health Resources and Services Administration, March 1999, U.S. Department of Health and Human Services, www.hrsa.gov; Financing Graduate Medical Education in a Changing Health Care Environment, Council on Graduate Medical Education / Fifteenth Report, Health Resources and Services Administration, December 2000, U.S. Department of Health and Human Services, www.hrsa.gov; Emily J. Cook et al, "Consolidated Appropriations Act Includes GME Support Provisions," National Law Review, January 15, 2021, www.natlawreview.com.

[203] Medicare Payment Advisory Commission / Public Meeting [transcript], October 3, 2019, www.medpac.gov; Report to the Congress / Medicare and the Health Care Delivery System, June 2019, Medicare Payment Advisory Commission, www.medpac.gov.

[204] "What is the Shortage Designation Management System?" Health Resources and Services Administration, accessed February 20, 2020, U.S. Department of Health and Human Services, www.bhw.hrsa.gov.

[205] The Future of the Nursing Workforce: National- and State-Level Projections, 2012-2025, Bureau of Health Workforce, National Center for Workforce Analysis, Health Resources and Services Administration, April 2017, U.S. Department of Health and Human Services, www.hrsa.gov; Supply and Demand Projections of the Nursing Workforce: 2014-2030, Bureau of Health Workforce, National Center for Workforce Analysis, Health Resources and Services Administration, July 21, 2017, U.S. Department of Health and Human Services, www.hrsa.gov.

[206] The Nation's Physician Workforce: Options for Balancing Supply and Requirements, National Academies Press, Institute of Medicine Committee on the U.S. Physician Supply, 1996, Institute of Medicine of the National Academies, www.nap.edu; "Health Care Workforce: Future Supply vs. Demand," Alliance for Health Reform (nka Alliance for Health Policy), April 2011, www.allhealthpolicy.org; OIG Determination of VHA's Occupational Staffing Shortages, FY 2019, Office of Inspector General, September 30, 2019, U.S. Department of Veterans Affairs, www.va.gov; "The Future of Nursing: Leading Change, Advancing Health," Committee on the Robert Wood Johnson

Foundation Initiative on the Future of Nursing at the Institute of Medicine, 2011, Institute of Medicine of the National Academies, www.nam.edu; "Out of Order, Out of Time – The State of the Nation's Health Workforce, 2013," Association of Academic Health Centers, 2013, www.aahcdc.org; "Health Care Workforce - Federal Investments in Training and the Availability of Data for Workforce Projections," United States Government Accountability Office, April 9, 2014, www.gao.gov; "Comprehensive Planning by HHS Needed to Meet National Needs," United States Government Accountability Office, December 2015, www.gao.gov; "Collecting Nursing Workforce Data," The Future of Nursing: Campaign for Action, Campaign for Action, January 28, 2020, Robert Wood Johnson Foundation, AARP Foundation and AARP, www.campaignforaction.org; Joanne Spetz, PhD FFAN et al, "Improving collection and use of interprofessional health workforce data: Progress and Peril," Nursing Outlook, March 2016, American Academy of Nursing and the Council for the Advancement of Nursing Science, www.nursingoutlook.org; Report to the Congress: Medicare and the Health Care Delivery System, June 2019, Medicare Payment Advisory Commission, www.medpac.gov.

[207] Long-Term Services and Supports: Direct Care Worker Demand Projections – 2015-2030, Health Resources and Services Administration, National Center for Health Workforce Analysis, March 2018, U.S. Department of Health and Human Services, www.bhw.hrsa.gov.

[208] Health Workforce Projections: Nursing Assistants and Home Health Aides, Bureau of Health Workforce, National Center for Workforce Analysis, Health Resources and Services Administration, September 2016, U.S. Department of Health and Human Services, www.hrsa.gov; Allied Health Workforce Projections, 2016-2030: Medical and Clinical Laboratory Technologists, Bureau of Health Workforce, National Center for Workforce Analysis, Health Resources and Services Administration, 2019, U.S. Department of Health and Human Services, www.hrsa.gov; Allied Health Workforce Projections, 2016-2030: Emergency Medical Technicians and Paramedics, Bureau of Health Workforce, National Center for Workforce Analysis, Health Resources and Services Administration, 2019, U.S. Department of Health and Human Services, www.hrsa.gov; Allied Health Workforce Projections, 2016-2030: Community Health Workers, Bureau of Health Workforce, National Center for Workforce Analysis, Health Resources and Services Administration, 2019, U.S. Department of Health and Human Services, www.hrsa.gov.

[209] Strategic Plan FY 2018-2022 – Strategic Objective 1.4: Strengthen and expand the healthcare workforce to meet America's diverse needs, accessed February 26, 2021, U.S. Department of Health and Human Services, www.hhs.gov; Strategic Plan: FY 2019-2022 - Goal 2: Foster a Health Care Workforce Able to Address Current and Emerging Needs, Health Resources and Service Administration, accessed January 26, 2021, U.S. Department of Health and Human Services, www.hrsa.gov.

[210] National Projections of Supply and Demand for Selected Behavioral Health Practitioners: 2013-2025, Bureau of Health Workforce, National Center for Workforce Analysis, Health Resources and Services Administration, November 2016, U.S. Department of Health and Human Services, www.hrsa.gov.

[211] Retooling for an Aging America / Building the Health Care Workforce, Committee on the Future Health Care Workforce for Older Americans, 2008, Institute of Medicine of the National Academies, www.nam.edu.

[212] "About Us," Bureau of Health Workforce, December 2020, U.S. Department of Health and Human Services, www.bhw.hrsa.gov; Records of the Health Resources and Services Administration [HRSA], National Archives, accessed February 26, 2021, www.archives.gov.

[213] Patient Protection and Affordable Care Act – Title V – Health Care Workforce, Subtitle B, Innovations in the Health Care Workforce, U.S.C. Sec. 5101 (Public Law 111-148), 2010.

[214] "The Future of Nursing: Leading Change, Advancing Health," Committee on the Robert Wood Johnson Foundation Initiative on the Future of Nursing at the Institute of Medicine, 2011, Institute of Medicine of the National Academies, www.nam.edu.

[215] Peter I. Buerhaus and Sheldon M. Retchin, "The Dormant National Health Care Workforce Commission Needs Congressional Funding to Fulfill Its Promise," Health Affairs, November 2013, Project HOPE, The People-to-People Health Foundation, Inc., www.healthaffairs.org; "GAO Calls for

Better Health Care Workforce Plan," University of Washington, January 14, 2016, www.washington.edu.
[216] Michael Grabell, Money Well Spent?: The Truth Behind the Trillion-Dollar Stimulus, the Biggest Economic Recovery Plan in History, Public Affairs, January 2012.
[217] About the Committee [Council on Graduate Medical Education], Federal Advisory Committees, U.S. Department of Health and Human Services, October 2020, www.hrsa.gov; Issue Brief: Graduate Medical Education, Medical Student Advocacy and Region Conference 2019, American Medical Association, 2019, www.ama-assn.org.
[218] Physician Workforce Policy Guidelines for the United States, 2000-2020, Council on Graduate Medical Education, Sixteenth Report, Health Resources and Services Administration, January 2005, U.S. Department of Health and Human Services, www.hrsa.gov; Towards the Development of a National Strategic Plan for Graduate Medical Education, Council on Graduate Medical Education, 23rd Report, Health Resources and Services Administration, April 2017, U.S. Department of Health and Human Services, www.hrsa.gov.
[219] Patient Protection and Affordable Care Act – Title V – Health Care Workforce, Subtitle B, Innovations in the Health Care Workforce, U.S.C. Sec. 5103 (Public Law 111-148), March 2010; "About the National Center for Health Workforce Analysis (NCHWA)," Health Resources and Services Administration, accessed November 27, 2020, U.S. Department of Health and Human Services, www.healthworkforceta.org.
[220] "National Center for Health Workforce Analysis, Health Workforce Technical Assistance Center" (located at the University at Albany, State University of New York), Health Resources and Services Administration, accessed November 27, 2020, U.S. Department of Health and Human Services, www.healthworkforceta.org.
[221] Physician Supply and Demand: Projections to 2020, Health Resources and Services Administration, October 2006, U.S. Department of Health and Human Services, www.hrsa.gov.
[222] 2018 National Sample Survey of Registered Nurses, Health Resources and Services Administration, January 2020, Bureau of Health Workforce, National Center for Health Workforce Analysis, U.S. Department of Health and Human Services, www.bhw.hrsa.gov; Nursing Workforce Survey Data (National Sample Survey of Registered Nurses), Health Resources & Services Administration, accessed February 27, 2021, www.healthdata.gov.
[223] Occupational Outlook Handbook: Healthcare Occupations, U.S. Bureau of Labor Statistics, September 4, 2019, U.S. Department of Labor, www.bls.gov; Occupational Outlook Handbook: Healthcare Occupations, U.S. Bureau of Labor Statistics, September 1, 2020, U.S. Department of Labor, www.bls.gov.
[224] Kerry Dooley Young, "Trump Executive Order Seeks Proposals on Medicare Pay for NPs, PAs," Medscape, October 3, 2019, www.medscape.com; Kevin B. O'Reilly, "How a presidential order threatens the physician-led care team," Payment & Delivery Models, October 29, 2019, American Medical Association, www.ama-assn.org; "AAFP Warns of More Harm in Scope-of-Practice Executive Order," American Academy of Family Practitioners, January 21, 2020, www.aafp.org.
[225] "National Survey Suggests U.S. May Not Be Facing a Doctor Shortage After All," TMC Health Policy Institute, November 12, 2019, Texas Medical Center, www.tmcnationspulse.org; Perri Morgan, PhD, PA-C, "Predicted shortages of physicians might even disappear if we fully account for PAs and NPs," Journal of the American Academy of PAs, October 2019, American Academy of PAs, www.jaapa.com.
[226] David I. Auerbach et al, "Implications of the Rapid Growth of the Nurse Practitioner Workforce in the U.S." Health Affairs, February 2020, Project HOPE, The People-to-People Health Foundation, Inc., www.healthaffairs.org.
[227] Emily Gudbranson, BA, Aaron Glickman, BA, Ezekiel J. Emanuel, MD, PhD, "Reassessing the Data on Whether a Physician Shortage Exists," Journal of the American Medical Association, May 16, 2017, American Medical Association, www.ama-assn.org.
[228] S. 299 – Geriatrics Workforce Improvement Act, 116th Congress (2019-2020), www.senate.gov; H.R. 647 – Palliative Care and Hospice Education and Training Act, 116th Congress (2019-2020),

www.congress.gov.

[229] S. 834 – Resident Physician Shortage Reduction Act of 2021, 117th Congress (2021-2022), www.congress.gov; Emily J. Cook et al, "Consolidated Appropriations Act Includes GME Support Provisions," National Law Review, January 15, 2021, www.natlawreview.com.

[230] Ida A. Brudnick, Congressional Salaries and Allowances: In Brief, CRS Report Prepared for Members and Committees of Congress, December 20, 2019, Congressional Research Service, www.crs.gov.

[231] Wendy R. Ginsburg, "Federal Advisory Committees: An Overview," CRS Report Prepared for Members and Committees of Congress, April 16, 2009, Congressional Research Service, www.crs.gov.

[232] "Welcome to the GSA Federal Advisory Committee Act (FACA) Database, Reporting Fiscal Year 2019 Government Totals," accessed March 10, 2020, U.S. General Services Administration, www.facadatabase.gov; "GSA Federal Advisory Committee Act (FACA) Database, Reporting Fiscal Year 2020 Government Totals," accessed December 5, 2020, U.S. General Services Administration, www.facadatabase.gov.

[233] All Agency Accounts, GSA Federal Advisory Committee Act (FACA) Database, accessed December 5, 2020, U.S. General Services Administration, www.facadatabase.gov.

[234] "HHS Organizational Chart," September 23, 2020, U.S. Department of Health and Human Services, www.hhs.gov; "Putting America's Health First – FY 2021 President's Budget for HHS," February 20, 2020, U.S. Department of Health and Human Services, www.hhs.gov.

[235] "GSA Federal Advisory Committee Act (FACA) Database, Reporting Fiscal Year 2020 Government Totals," accessed December 5, 2020, U.S. General Services Administration, www.facadatabase.gov.

CHAPTER SEVEN

[236] "Rural Americans at higher risk of death from five leading causes," Press Release, Centers for Disease Control and Prevention, January 12, 2017, U.S. Department of Health and Human Services, www.cdc.gov.

[237] "Analysis Shows One-in-Five U.S. Rural Hospitals at High Risk of Closing Unless Financial Situation Improves," Navigant Consulting, Inc., February 20, 2019, www.navigant.com; Rural Hospitals at Risk of Closing, Center for Healthcare Quality and Payment Reform, January 2021, www.ruralhospitals.org.

[238] Jill J. Ashman, Ph.D. et al, Emergency Department Visits Among Adults Aged 60 and Over: United States, 2014-2017," Centers for Disease Control and Prevention, June 2020, U.S. Department of Health and Human Services, www.cdc.gov.

[239] 2018 Survey of America's Physicians, Practice Patterns and Perspectives, conducted by Merritt Hawkins and AMN Healthcare, September 2018, The Physicians Foundation, www.physiciansfoundation.org; Medicaid Acceptance Rates by Coverage Type, The Medicaid and CHIP Payment and Access Commission (MACPAC), an advisory committee of the United States Congress, January 24, 2019, www.macpac.gov; Kayla Holgash and Martha Heberlein, "Physician Acceptance of New Medicaid Patients: What Matters and What Doesn't," Health Affairs, April 10, 2019, Project HOPE, The People-to-People Health Foundation, Inc., www.healthaffairs.org.

[240] Care Redesign Survey: To Improve Chronic Disease Care, Change the Payment Model, New England Journal of Medicine Catalyst Insights Council, September 5, 2019, Massachusetts Medical Society, www.catalyst.nejm.org.

[241] "Delayed Cancer Screenings," Epic Health Research Network, May 4, 2020, www.ehrn.org; "Routine Chronic Disease Screenings and Oncology Biomarker Tests Plummet During COVID-19," Komodo Health, April 2020, www.komodohealth.com; Ronald C. Chen, MD, MPH et al, "Association of Cancer Screening Deficit in the United States With the COVID-19 Pandemic, JAMA Oncology, April 29, 2021, American Medical Association, www.jamanetwork.org.

[242] Elizabeth A. Carter, "Annual Wellness Visits among Medicare Advantage Enrollees: Trends, Differences by Race and Ethnicity, and Association with Preventive Service Use," AARP Public Policy Institute, May 2019, AARP, www.aarp.org/ppi.

[243] David M. Levine, MD, MPH, MA et al, "Characteristics of Americans With Primary Care and Changes Over Time, 2002-2015," JAMA of Internal Medicine, March 2020, American Medical Association, www.jamainternalmedicine.com.

[244] Occupational Outlook Handbook: Healthcare Occupations, U.S. Bureau of Labor Statistics, September 1, 2020, U.S. Department of Labor, www.bls.gov.

[245] Timothy M. Snavely, "A brief economic analysis of the looming nursing shortage in the United States," Nursing Economic$, March 1, 2016, www.nursingeconomics.net.

[246] "Targeted Solutions Tool (TST) - Handoff Communications," Joint Commission Center for Transforming Healthcare, accessed November 18, 2020, The Joint Commission, www.jointcommission.org.

[247] Vernon W. Lin et al, "U.S. Social Worker Workforce Report Card: Forecasting Nationwide Shortages," Journal of Social Work, November 2015, www.research; Occupational Outlook Handbook: Healthcare Occupations, U.S. Bureau of Labor Statistics, September 1, 2020, U.S. Department of Labor, www.bls.gov.

[248] Households by Size: 1960 to Present, U.S. Census Bureau, December 2020, U.S. Department of Commerce, www.census.gov.

[249] Donald Redfoot et al, "The Aging of the Baby Boom and the Growing Care Gap: A Look at Future Declines in the Availability of Family Caregivers," Insight on the Issues, AARP Public Policy Institute, August 2013, AARP, www.aarp.org/ppi.

[250] Caregiving in the U.S., AARP and the National Alliance for Caregiving, May 2020, www.AARP.org; "Caregiver Statistics: Demographics," Family Caregiver Alliance, April 17, 2019, National Center on Caregiving, www.caregiver.org.

[251] Maria T. Carney et al, "Elder Orphans Hiding in Plain Sight: A Growing Vulnerable Population," Current Gerontology and Geriatrics Research, October 2016, www.hindawi.com; Table 2. Projected Age Groups and Sex Composition of the Population, Projections for the United States: 2017-2060, U.S. Census Bureau, 2016, U.S. Department of Commerce, www.census.gov.

[252] Donald Redfoot et al, "The Aging of the Baby Boom and the Growing Care Gap: A Look at Future Declines in the Availability of Family Caregivers," Insight on the Issues, AARP Public Policy Institute, August 2013, AARP, www.aarp.org/ppi.

[253] Occupational Outlook Handbook: Healthcare Occupations, U.S. Bureau of Labor Statistics, February 28, 2021, U.S. Department of Labor, www.bls.gov; Stephen Campbell et al, "Caring for the Future: The Power and Potential of America's Direct Care Workforce," PHI (formerly Paraprofessional Healthcare Institute), January 21, 2020, www.phinational.org.

[254] Projections and Implications for Housing, A Growing Population: Older Households 2015-2035, Joint Center for Housing Studies of Harvard University, 2016, Harvard College, www.jchs.harvard.edu.

[255] "What is the Lifetime Risk of Needing and Receiving Long-Term Services and Supports?," ASPE Research Brief, Office of Disability, Aging and Long-Term Care Policy, HHS Office of the Assistant Secretary for Planning and Evaluation, April 2019, U.S. Department of Health and Human Services, www.aspe.hhs.gov; "2020 Alzheimer's Disease Facts and Figures," Alzheimer's & Dementia, Journal of the Alzheimer's Association, March 2020, Alzheimer's Association, www.alz.org.

[256] Charlene Harrington et al, "Appropriate Nurse Staffing Levels for U.S. Nursing Homes," Health Services Insights, July 29, 2020, www.journals.sagepub.com.

[257] Jordan Rau, "Like a Ghost Town: Erratic Nursing Home Staffing Revealed Through New Records," Kaiser Health News, July 13, 2018, www.khn.org; Occupational Outlook Handbook: Healthcare Occupations, U.S. Bureau of Labor Statistics, September 1, 2020, U.S. Department of Labor, www.bls.gov.

[258] "Alzheimer's / Dementia Care Costs: Home Care, Adult Day Care, Assisted Living & Nursing Homes," Dementia Care Central, October 23, 2019, www.dementiacarecentral.com; "2020 Alzheimer's Disease Facts and Figures," Alzheimer's & Dementia, Journal of the Alzheimer's Association, March 2020, Alzheimer's Association, www.alz.org; "Cost of Care," Genworth Financial, Inc., August 2020, www.genworth.com.

CHAPTER EIGHT

[259] Paul Jolly, "Medical Education In the United States, 1960-1987," Health Affairs DataWatch, 1988,

Project HOPE, The People-to-People Health Foundation, Inc., www.healthaffairs.org; Mary A. Fruen, Medical Education and Societal Needs: A Planning Report for the Health Professions, Chapter 8, How the Medical Student Finances Educational Expenses, Institute of Medicine, National Institutes of Health, 1983, U.S. Department of Health and Human Services, www.ncbi.nlm.nih.gov; Table 332.45 Percentage of graduate degree completers with student loan debt and average cumulative amount owed, National Center for Education Statistics, January 2018, U.S. Department of Education, www.nces.ed.gov; "An Updated Look at Attendance Cost and Medical Student Debt at U.S. Medical Schools," Analysis in Brief, August 2017, Association of American Medical Colleges, www.aamc.org; Tuition and Student Fees for First-Year Students, AAMC Tuition and Student Fees Questionnaire, February 2020, Association of American Medical Colleges, www.aamc.org; "Trends in Cost and Debt at U.S. Medical Schools Using a New Measure of Medical School Cost of Attendance," Analysis in Brief, July 2012, Association of American Medical Colleges, www.aamc.org; Medical Student Education: Debt, Costs, and Loan Repayment Fact Card, Association of American Medical Colleges, October 2018, www.aamc.org.

[260] Peter Densen, MD, "Challenges and Opportunities Facing Medical Education," Transactions of the American Clinical and Climatological Association, January 2010, American Clinical and Climatological Association, www.ncbi.nlm.nih.gov.

[261] "Code set differences (ICD-10-CM/PCS)," Centers for Disease Prevention and Control, accessed December 13, 2020, U.S. Department of Health and Human Services, www.cdc.gov.

[262] 2018 Survey of America's Physicians: Practice, Patterns and Perspectives, Physicians Foundation, September 2018, www.physiciansfoundation.org; Christine Sinsky, MD et al, "Allocation of Physician Time in Ambulatory Practice: A Time and Motion Study in 4 Specialties," Annals of Internal Medicine, December 6, 2016, American College of Physicians, www.annals.org; Taking Action Against Clinician Burnout: A Systems Approach to Professional Well-Being, Committee on Systems Approaches to Improve Patient Care by Supporting Clinician Well-Being, 2019, National Academy of Medicine, www.nap.edu; Scott W. Yates, MD, MBA MS, FACP, "Physician Stress and Burnout," The American Journal of Medicine, February 2020, Alliance for Academic Internal Medicine, www.amjmed.com; Physician Compensation Report 2020, Medscape, May 14, 2020, www.medscape.com.

[263] Melissa Thomasson, "Health Insurance in the United States," Economic History Association, April 17, 2003, www.eh.net; U.S. Health Care Coverage and Spending, Congressional Research Service, January 26, 2021, U.S. Congress, www.crsreports.congress.gov.

[264] Chapin White and Christopher Whaley, "Prices Paid to Hospitals by Private Health Plans Are High Relative to Medicare and Vary Widely," Rand Corporation, 2019, www.rand.org; Daria Pelech, An Analysis of Private-Sector Prices for Physicians' Services, Working Paper Series, January 2018, Congressional Budget Office, www.cbo.gov.

[265] Emily Gee and Topher Spiro, "Excess Administrative Costs Burden the U.S. Health Care System," Center for American Progress (citing Centers for Medicare and Medicaid Services data), April 8, 2019, www.americanprogress.org; David U. Himmelstein, MD et al, "Health Care Administrative Costs in the United States and Canada, 2017," Annals of Internal Medicine, January 21, 2020, American College of Physicians, www.annals.org.

[266] Taking Action Against Clinician Burnout: A Systems Approach to Professional Well-Being, Committee on Systems Approaches to Improve Patient Care by Supporting Clinician Well-Being, 2019, National Academy of Medicine, www.nap.edu; Leslie Kane, MA and Wendy K. Dean, MD, "Medscape National Physician Burnout & Suicide Report 2020: The Generational Divide," Medscape, January 15, 2020, www.medscape.com; Leslie Kane, MA, MD, "Death by 1000 Cuts: Medscape National Physician Burnout & Suicide Report 2021," Medscape, January 22, 2021, www.medscape.com; Nikitha K. Menon, BA et al, "Association of Physician Burnout With Suicidal Ideation and Medical Errors," JAMA Network Open, December 9, 2020, www.jamanetwork.com.

[267] 2018 Survey of America's Physicians: Practice, Patterns and Perspectives, Physicians Foundation, September 2018, www.physiciansfoundation.org; Patricia Wendling, "More than one in three cardiologists burned out, many ready to bolt," MDEdge – Cardiology, March 28 2020, American College

of Cardiology, www.mdedge.com; Position Paper: The Business Case for Humanity in Healthcare, National Taskforce for Humanity in Healthcare, April 2018, Institute for Healthcare Excellence, www.healthcareexcellence.org; Scott W. Yates, MD, MBA MS, FACP, "Physician Stress and Burnout," The American Journal of Medicine, February 2020, Alliance for Academic Internal Medicine, www.amjmed.com; Physician Workload Survey 2018, Locum Story, August 1, 2018, www.locumstory.com; Lesly A. Kelly, PhD, RN, FAAN et al, "Impact of nurse burnout on organizational and position turnover," Nursing Outlook, January/February 2021, www.sciencedirect.com; Lotte N. Dyrbye, MD, MHPE et al, "Burnout and satisfaction with work-life integration among PAs relative to other workers," Journal of the American Academy of Physician Assistants, May 2020, American Academy of Physician Assistants, www.journals.lww.com.

[268] 2018 Survey of America's Physicians: Practice, Patterns and Perspectives, Physicians Foundation, September 2018, www.physiciansfoundation.org; The Future of Healthcare – A National Survey of Physicians, The Doctors Company, 2018, www.thedoctors.com.

[269] Position Paper: The Business Case for Humanity in Healthcare, National Taskforce for Humanity in Healthcare, April 2018, Institute for Healthcare Excellence, www.healthcareexcellence.org; Sara Berg, "How much physician burnout is costing your organization," American Medical Association, October 11, 2018, www.ama-assn.org; Rikinkumar S. Patel et al, "A Review on Strategies to Manage Physician Burnout," The Cureus Journal of Medical Science, June 3, 2019, www.cureus.com; Scott W. Yates, MD, MBA MS, FACP, "Physician Stress and Burnout," The American Journal of Medicine, February 2020, Alliance for Academic Internal Medicine, www.amjmed.com; Sara Berg, "At Stanford, physician burnout costs at least $7.75 million a year." American Medical Association, November 17, 2017, www.ama-assn.org.

[270] Shasha Han, MS et al, "Estimating the Attributable Cost of Physician Burnout in the United States," Annals of Internal Medicine, June 4, 2019, American College of Physicians, www.annals.org; Scott W. Yates, MD, MBA MS, FACP, "Physician Stress and Burnout," The American Journal of Medicine, February 2020, www.amjmed.com.

[271] Leslie Kane, MA and Wendy K. Dean, MD, "Medscape National Physician Burnout & Suicide Report 2020: The Generational Divide," Medscape, January 15, 2020, www.medscape.com; Leslie Kane, MA, "Death by 1000 Cuts: Medscape National Physician Burnout & Suicide Report 2021, January 21, 2021, www.medscape.com; 2018 Survey of America's Physicians: Practice, Patterns and Perspectives, Physicians Foundation, September 2018, www.physiciansfoundation.org; 2020 Survey of America's Physicians/COVID-19 Impact Edition, Physicians Foundation, August 2020, www.physiciansfoundation.org.

[272] Christine A. Sinsky, MD et al, "Professional Satisfaction and the Career Plans of U.S. Physicians," Mayo Clinic Proceedings, November 2017, Mayo Clinic, www.mayoclinicproceedings.org; 2019 Physician Burnout Survey: Results show growing crisis in medicine, August 12, 2019, Medical Economics, www.medicaleconomics.com; "One in five surgeons set to retire early due to physical toll," CMR Surgical, September 15, 2019, www.cmrsurgical.com; RNnetwork 2018 Portrait of a Modern Nurse Survey, RNnetwork, December 12, 2018, www.rnnetwork.com; Physicians Still Miserable: Seven Solutions to Address Burnout, Geneia, LLC, November 19, 2019, www.geneia.com; The Future of Healthcare – A National Survey of Physicians, The Doctors Company, 2018, www.thedoctors.com; 2018 Survey of America's Physicians: Practice, Patterns and Perspectives, Physicians Foundation, September 2018, www.physiciansfoundation.org; Putting Profits Before Patients: Provider Perspectives on Health Insurance Barriers That Harm Patients, The Alliance for the Adoption of Innovations of Medicine, October 2018, www.aimedalliance.org.

[273] Meeting Brief – Updates to the methods used to assess the adequacy of Medicare payment for physician and other health professional services, Medicare Payment Advisory Commission (MedPAC), October 3-4, 2019, www.medpac.gov; Report: Demand for Specialist Physicians Driving Physician Recruitment, Merritt Hawkins, an AMN Healthcare Company, July 8, 2019, www.amnhealthcare.com; Leslie Kane, MA, Medscape Physician Compensation Report 2020, Medscape, May 14, 2020, www.medscape.com.

[274] Physician Workload Survey 2018, Locum Story, August 1, 2018, www.locumstory.com; 2019 Physician Burnout Survey: Results show growing crisis in medicine, August 12, 2019, Medical Economics, www.medicaleconomics.com; Taking Action Against Clinician Burnout: A Systems Approach to Professional Well-Being, Committee on Systems Approaches to Improve Patient Care by Supporting Clinician Well-Being, 2019, National Academy of Medicine, www.nap.edu.
[275] "AMA analysis shows most physicians work outside of private practice," Press Release, May 5, 2021, American Medical Association, www.ama-assn.org; Carol K. Kane, PhD, "Updated Data on Physician Practice Arrangements: For the First Time, Fewer Physicians are Owners Than Employees, AMA Economic and Health Policy Research, May 2019, American Medical Association, www.ama-assn.org.
[276] "What is a hospitalist? Hospital Medicine 101," Society of Hospital Medicine, accessed April 8, 2020, www.hospitalmedicine.org; Stephanie Stephens, "The Rise of Hospitalists—and What Comes Next," Health eCareers, December 17, 2019, www.healthecareers.com; Sohail Abdul Salim et al, "Impact of hospitalists on the efficiency of inpatient care and patient satisfaction: A systematic review and meta-analysis," Journal of Community Hospital Internal Medicine Perspectives, March 2019, Greater Baltimore Medical Center, www.tandfonline.com.
[277] Medicare Payment Advisory Commission Public Meeting, Medicare Payment Advisory Commission (MedPAC), October 3, 2019, www.medpac.gov.
[278] Coleen Kivlahan, MD, MSPH et al, "Calculating Primary Care Panel Size," UC Center for Health Quality and Innovation, January 2017, University of California, www.ucop.edu.
[279] Melanie Raffoul et al, "A Primary Care Panel Size of 2500 is Neither Accurate nor Reasonable," Journal of the American Board of Family Medicine, July-August 2016, American Board of Family Medicine, www.jabfm.org
[280] 2018 Survey of America's Physicians: Practice, Patterns and Perspectives, Physicians Foundation, September 2018, www.physiciansfoundation.org; 90th Annual Physician Report, Medical Economics, April 17, 2019, www.medicaleconomics.com.
[281] Rob Lamberts, MD, "Difference between concierge and direct care," Medical Economics, February 18, 2019, www.medicaleconomics.com; "Medical Q&A: Concierge care is not for everyone; that's the point," Sarasota Herald-Tribune, November 5, 2019, www.heraldtribune.com; "National Estimates on Growth and Numbers in 2018-2019," Concierge Medicine Today, LLC, June/July 2019, www.conciergemedicinetoday.org; "What is concierge care? See how the retainer-based care model is filling care gaps and driving new revenue," Advisory Board, July 8, 2014, www.advisory.com; "Here's what patients most often want to know about concierge medicine," Specialdocs Consultants, accessed May 11, 2020, www.specialdocs.com; 2019 State of the Concierge Medicine Physician Survey, Specialdocs Consultants, 2019, www.specialdocs.com.
[282] "Opting Out of Medicare," DCP Frontier, accessed August 1, 2020, www.dpcfrontier.com; "Is my test, item, or service covered? / Concierge care," Centers for Medicare and Medicaid Services, accessed May 12, 2020, U.S. Department of Health and Human Services, www.cms.gov.
[283] Philip M. Eskew, DO, JD, MBA and Kathleen Klink, MD, "Direct Primary Care: Practice Distribution and Cost Across the Nation," Journal of the American Board of Family Medicine, November 2015, American Board of Family Medicine, www.jabfm.org; 2018 Direct Primary Care (DPC) Study, American Academy of Family Physicians, March 2018, www.aafp.org; Rob Lamberts, MD, "Difference between concierge and direct care," Medical Economics, February 18, 2019, www.medicaleconomics.com; "Letter to Administrator Verma responding to CMS RFI on Direct Provider Contracting," American Academy of Family Physicians, May 25, 2018, www.aafp.org.
[284] Ambulatory Care Use and Physician Office Visits, Centers for Disease Control and Prevention, National Center for Health Statistics, January 2019, U.S. Department of Health and Human Services, www.cdc.gov.
[285] 2020 Profile of Older Americans, Administration for Community Living, Administration on Aging, May 2020, U.S. Department of Health and Human Services, www.acl.gov.
[286] "Opt Out Affidavits," Centers for Medicare and Medicaid Services (CMS), February 11, 2020, U.S.

Department of Health and Human Services, www.cms.gov; Cristina Boccuti et al, Primary Care Physicians Accepting Medicare: A Snapshot, The Henry J. Kaiser Family Foundation, October 30, 2015, www.kff.org; 2018 Survey of America's Physicians: Practice, Patterns and Perspectives, Physicians Foundation, September 2018, www.physiciansfoundation.org; Kayla Holgash and Martha Heberlein, "Physician Acceptance of New Medicaid Patients," Medicaid and CHIP Payment and Access Commission, January 24, 2019, U.S. Department of Health and Human Services, www.macpac.gov.

[287] "Dental Benefits and Medicaid," Health Policy Institute, accessed April 20, 2021, American Dental Association, www.ada.org.

CHAPTER NINE

[288] Barry D. Weiss, MD, Health literacy and patient safety: Help patients understand – Manual for clinicians – Second edition, American Medical Association Foundation and American Medical Association, May 2007, www.amafoundation.org; "How Health Literate Are You?," The PEW Charitable Trusts, October 14, 2020, www.pewtrusts.org.

[289] Health Literacy Data Map, University of North Carolina at Chapel Hill, January 23, 2021, www.healthliteracymap.unc.edu.

[290] "The Federal Government Supports Health Literacy Research!" Centers for Disease Control and Prevention, email received from no-reply@emailupdates.cdc.gov, January 8, 2020.

[291] "Visualizing Patterns and Trends of 25 years of Published Health Literacy Research," HLRP: Health Literacy Research and Practice, October 2017, www.healio.com.

[292] Health Literacy – A Prescription to End Confusion, Committee on Health Literacy, Board on Neuroscience and Behavioral Health, 2004, Institute of Medicine of the National Academies, www.nam.edu.

[293] Donald Rubin, PhD, Consultant to Creative Thinkers, LLC, A Health Literacy Report: Analysis of 2016 BRFSS Health Literacy Data, Office of the Associate Director for Communication, Centers for Disease Control and Prevention, 2016, U.S. Department of Health and Human Services, www.cdc.gov.

[294] Adam E. M. Eltorai et al, "Readability of Patient Education Materials on the American Association for Surgery Trauma Website," Archives of Trauma Research, June 2014, Kashan University of Medical Sciences, www.archtrauma.com; Faith Lagay, PhD, "Reducing the Effects of Low Health Literacy," AMA Journal of Ethics, accessed November 29, 2020, www.journalofethics.ama-assn.org; Barry D. Weiss, MD, Health literacy and patient safety: Help patients understand – Manual for clinicians – Second edition, American Medical Association Foundation and American Medical Association, May 2007, www.amafoundation.org; Russell Rothman, MD, "Do the Math: Improving Health Literacy," The NEJM Catalyst event "Expanding the Bounds of Care Delivery: Integrating Mental, Social, and Physical Health," held at Vanderbilt University Medical Center, New England Journal of Medicine, January 25, 2018, Massachusetts Medical Society, www.catalyst.nejm.org.

[295] "Federal and State Websites Flunk COVID-19 Reading-Level Review," Dartmouth Neukom Institute for Computational Science, August 18, 2020, Dartmouth College, www.dartmouth.edu; Vishala Mishra, MBBS and Joseph P. Dexter, PhD, "Comparison of Readability of Official Public Health Information About COVID-19 on Websites of International Agencies and the Governments of 15 Countries," JAMA Network Open, August 18, 2020, American Medical Association, www.jamanetwork.com.

[296] Mark Kutner et al, The Health Literacy of America's Adults – Results from the 2003 National Assessment of Adult Literacy, American Institutes for Research, National Center for Education Statistics, Institute of Education Sciences, September 2006, U.S. Department of Education, www.nces.ed.gov.

[297] National Action Plan to Improve Health Literacy, Office of Disease Prevention and Health Promotion, May 2010, U.S. Department of Health and Human Services, www.health.gov.

[298] "Health Literate Care Model – A Universal Precautions Approach," Office of Disease Prevention and Health Promotion, January 16, 2020, U.S. Department of Health and Human Services, www.health.gov; "Health Literacy Online – A Guide for Simplifying the User Experience," Office of Disease Prevention and Health Promotion, December 31, 2019, U.S. Department of Health and Human Services, www.health.gov.

[299] "Comprehensive Summary of Objectives: Health Communication," Healthy People 2010, Office of Disease Prevention and Health Promotion, 2000, U.S. Department of Health and Human Services, www.health.gov; "Health Communication and Health Information Technology," Healthy People 2020, Office of Disease Prevention and Health Promotion, 2010, U.S. Department of Health and Human Services, www.health.gov.
[300] Building the Case for Health Literacy – Proceedings of a Workshop, Roundtable on Health Literacy, Board on Population Health and Public Health Practice, November 15, 2017, National Academies of Sciences, Engineering and Medicine, www.nap.edu.
[301] "Organizations & Committees / U.S. Department of Health and Human Services' Health Literacy Web Pages," Centers for Disease Control and Prevention, October 23, 2019, U.S. Department of Health and Human Services, www.cdc.gov.
[302] "Health Literacy," The Office of Disease Prevention and Health Promotion, accessed December 3, 2020, U.S. Department of Health and Human Services, www.health.gov; "Health Literacy," Agency for Healthcare Research and Quality, September 2020, U.S. Department of Health and Human Services, www.ahrq.gov; "Health literacy," Centers for Disease Control and Prevention, November 30, 2020, U.S. Department of Health and Human Services, www.cdc.gov.
[303] "Health Literacy Activities by State," Centers for Disease Control and Prevention, December 2020, U.S. Department of Health and Human Services, www.cdc.gov. (And it was Worchester State University's www.centralmasshealthliteracy.org site that misspelled *literacy* and now appears to be closed down.)
[304] "AHRQ Launches New App Challenge to Advance Care Through Patient Self-Assessments," Agency for Healthcare Research and Quality, August 13, 2018, U.S. Department of Health and Human Services, www.ahrq.gov; The Growing Value of Digital Health, Institute Report, November 7, 2017, IQVIA, www.iqvia.com; David W. Bates et al, "Health apps and health policy: what is needed?" JAMA Network Open, November 20, 2018, American Medical Association, www.jamanetwork.com; William J. Gordon, "Beyond validation: getting health apps into clinical practice," npj digital medicine, February 3, 2020, Nature Research, www.nature.com.
[305] AHRQ Health Literacy Universal Precautions Toolkit, Second Edition, Agency for Healthcare Research and Quality, January 2015, accessed March 2, 2021, U.S. Department of Health and Human Services, www.ahrq.gov; Barry D. Weiss, MD, Health literacy and patient safety: Help patients understand – Manual for clinicians – Second edition, American Medical Association Foundation and American Medical Association, May 2007, www.amafoundation.org; Committee on Patient Safety and Quality Improvement and Committee on Health Care for Underserved Women, "Health Literacy to Promote Quality of Care," Committee Opinion, October 2016 (reaffirmed 2019), The American College of Obstetricians and Gynecologists; Health Literacy and Patient Engagement, Advisory Committee on Training in Primary Care Medicine and Dentistry, Twelfth Annual Report of the Secretary of the United States Department of Health and Human Services and the Congress of the United States, September 2015, U.S. Department of Health and Human Services, www.hrsa.gov; Building the Case for Health Literacy – Proceedings of a Workshop, Roundtable on Health Literacy, Board on Population Health and Public Health Practice, November 15, 2017, National Academies of Sciences, Engineering and Medicine, www.nap.edu; Health Literacy: Hidden Barriers and Practical Strategies, Agency for Healthcare Research and Quality, September 2020, U.S. Department of Health and Human Services, www.ahrq.gov; Health Literacy – Find Training, Centers for Disease Control and Prevention, December 14, 2020, U.S. Department of Health and Human Services, www.cdc.gov; Sample Action Plan to Improve Health Literacy, Office of Disease Prevention and Health Promotion, 2007, accessed August 29, 2019, U.S. Department of Health and Human Services, www.health.gov; Improving America's Oral Health Literacy, Delta Dental Institute, February 13, 2020, www.deltadentalinstitute.com; "Patient Safety Essentials Toolkit: Ask Me 3," Institute for Healthcare Improvement, 2019, www.ihi.org.
[306] Patient Self Determination Act of 1990 (H.R. 4449, 101st Congress (1989-1990), 42 CFR § 489.100-104; Kuldeep N. Yadav et al, "Approximately One In Three US Adults Completes Any Type Of Advance Directive for End-Of-Life Care," Project HOPE, The People-to-People Health Foundation, Inc., July 2017,

Health Affairs, www.healthaffairs.org; Jaya K. Rao, MD et al, "Completion of Advance Directives Among U.S. Consumers," American Journal of Preventive Medicine, January 2014, American College of Preventive Medicine and the Association for Prevention Teaching and Research, www.ajpmonline.org.
[307] "Mission and Budget," Agency for Healthcare Research and Quality, February 2020, U.S. Department of Health and Human Services, www.ahrq.gov.
[308] This is the definition of health literacy accepted for well over two decades, by the World Health Organization, the National Library of Medicine, the Healthy People campaigns of 2010 and 2020, the 2010 Affordable Care Act, the Institute of Medicine, the Centers for Disease Control and Prevention, the Agency for Healthcare Research and Quality, the National Institutes of Health, and countless advocacy groups and private enterprises.
[309] Secretary's Advisory Committee Report on Approaches to Healthy People 2030, The Secretary's Advisory Committee for 2030: Committee Reports and Meetings, April 27, 2017, Healthy People 2030, U.S. Department of Health and Human Services, www.healthypeople.gov, citing National Action Plan to Improve Health Literacy, Office of Disease Prevention and Health Promotion, May 2010, U.S. Department of Health and Human Services, www.hhs.gov; About Health Literacy, Agency for Healthcare Research and Quality, accessed March 12, 2021, U.S. Department of Health and Human Services, www.ahrq.gov; Understanding Health Literacy, Centers for Disease Control and Prevention, October 22, 2019, U.S. Department of Health and Human Services, www.cdc.gov.
[310] Secretary's Advisory Committee on National Health Promotion and Disease Prevention Objectives for 2030, Report #2, Recommendations for Developing Objectives, Setting Priorities, Identifying Data Needs, and Involving Stakeholders for Healthy People 2030, January 20, 2018, U.S. Department of Health and Human Services, www.healthypeople.gov; "Healthy People 2030 Proposes Redefining Health Literacy," Healthy People 2030 Health Communication and Health Information Technology Workgroup, Health Literacy Definition Committee, June 26, 2019, Agency for Healthcare Research and Quality, Centers for Disease Control and Prevention, U.S. Department of Health and Human Services, www.cdc.gov.
[311] Building the Case for Health Literacy – Proceedings of a Workshop, Roundtable on Health Literacy, Board on Population Health and Public Health Practice, November 15, 2017, National Academies of Sciences, Engineering and Medicine, www.nap.edu.
[312] Federal Register: Solicitation for Written Comments on an Updated Health Literacy Definition for Healthy People 2030, Office of Disease Prevention and Health Promotion, Office of the Assistant Secretary for Health, Office of the Secretary, June 4, 2019, Federal Register, www.federalregister.gov.
[313] Reframing Health Literacy for the Next Decade of Healthy People and History of Health Literacy Definitions, Office of Disease Prevention and Health Promotion, October 16, 2020, U.S. Department of Health and Human Services, www.health.gov.
[314] "Increase the health literacy of the population – HC/HIT-R01 – Status: Research," Healthy People 2030, Office of Disease Prevention and Health Promotion, December 8, 2020, U.S. Department of Health and Human Services, www.healthypeople.gov.
[315] Healthy People 2030 Questions & Answers, Office of Disease Prevention and Health Promotion, accessed June 10, 2021, U.S. Department of Health and Human Services, www.health.gov; "A riddle wrapped in a mystery inside an enigma." Winston Churchill.

CHAPTER ELEVEN

[316] Jo Kline, JD, The 60-Minute Guide to Health Literacy – A common sense approach to informed medical decision making, Providentia Publishing, 2017, www.amazon.com.
[317] A nod to Mark Twain. *"The difference between the almost right word and the right word is really a large matter. 'Tis the difference between the lightning bug and the lightning."*

CHAPTER TWELVE

[318] Tyler Barreto, MD et al, "Family Physicians Practicing High-Volume Obstetric Care have Recently Dropped by One-Half," American Family Physician, Graham Center Policy One-Pager, June 2017, American Academy of Family Physicians, www.aafp.org.
[319] Canterbury v. Spence, 464 F. 2d 772. United States Court of Appeals, D.C. Circuit Court, May 19,

1972; Barry D. Weiss, MD, Health literacy and patient safety: Help patients understand – Manual for clinicians, Second Edition, American Medical Association Foundation and American Medical Association, May 2007, www.ama-assn.org.

[320] "Hidden Hazards: Closing the Care Gap Between Physicians and Patients With Multiple Chronic Conditions," Regina Corso Consulting, February 2018, Quest Diagnostics, www.questdiagnostics.com.

[321] Glyn Elwyn, MB BCh, PhD, "Integrating Shared Decision-Making and Interprofessional Education," The Josiah Macy Jr. Foundation, May 2014, www.macyfoundation.org; Alexis M. Stoner, MPH, PhD et al, "The Other 45: Improving Patients' Chronic Disease Self-management and Medical Students' Communication Skills," Journal of the American Osteopathic Association, November 2018, American Osteopathic Association, www.jaoa.org.

[322] Marie-Anne Durand et al, "Shared decision making imbedded in the undergraduate medical curriculum: A scoping review," PLOS ONE, November 14, 2018, www.journals.plos.org.

[323] "The SHARE Approach," Agency for Healthcare Research & Quality, July 2014, accessed December 21, 2020, U.S. Department of Health and Human Services, www.ahrq.gov.

[324] "Fact Sheet: Beneficiary Engagement and Incentives Models: Shared Decision Making Model," Centers for Medicare and Medicaid Services, December 8, 2016, U.S. Department of Health and Human Services, www.cms.gov; "CMS Cancels Shared Decision-Making Models Due to Planning Issues," Xtelligent Media, February 6, 2018, www.patientengagementhit.com (link to CMS explanatory CMS press release not available).

[325] "Hidden Hazards: Closing the Care Gap Between Physicians and Patients With Multiple Chronic Conditions," Regina Corso Consulting, February 2018, Quest Diagnostics, www.questdiagnostics.com.

[326] Surveys of Trust in the U.S. Health Care System," American Board of Internal Medicine Foundation, May 21, 2021, www.buildingtrust.org; The Power of the Patient Voice: How Health Care Organizations Empower Patients and Improve Care Delivery, NEJM Catalyst, March 15, 2021, Massachusetts Medical Society, www.catalyst.nejm.org; Ana C. DeRoo, MD, MSc et al, "High-risk surgery among older adults: Not-quite shared decision-making," Surgery, March 10, 2021, Society of University Surgeons, Central Surgical Association, American Association of Endocrine Surgeons, www.sciencedirect.com; Laurie E. Gaspar et al, "The patient experience with shared decision-making in lung cancer: A survey of patients, significant others or care givers," Patient Experience Journal, April 2018, www.pxjournal.org; John T. James et al, "Informed consent, shared-decision making and a reasonable patient's wishes based on a cross-sectional, national survey in the USA using a hypothetical scenario," BMJ Open, July 12, 2019, www.bjmopen.bmj.com; "The SHARE Approach," Agency for Healthcare Research & Quality, July 2014, accessed December 21, 2020, U.S. Department of Health and Human Services, www.ahrq.gov; "Care Coordination Improving, Technology and 24/7 Access Not Widely Available, and Preventive Primary Care Critically Lacking," Council of Accountable Physician Practices (CAPP), June 15, 2016, www.accountablecaredoctors.org; Jordan R. Covvey, "Barriers and facilitators to shared decision-making in oncology: a systematic review of the literature," Supportive Care in Cancer, February 8, 2019, Multinational Association of Supportive Care in Cancer, www.springer.com.

[327] Jane C. Weeks, MD et al, "Patients' Expectations about Effects of Chemotherapy for Advanced Cancer," The New England Journal of Medicine, October 25, 2012, Massachusetts Medical Society, www.nejm.org; Andrew S. Epstein et al, "Discussions of Life Expectancy and Changes in Illness Understanding in Patients with Advanced Cancer," Journal of Clinical Oncology, September 27, 2016, American Society of Clinical Oncology, www.ascopubs.org.

[328] Jacqueline M. Garonzik-Wang, MD, PhD et al, "Missing Consent Forms in the Preoperative Area – A Single-Center Assessment of the Scope of the Problem and Its Downstream Effects," Journal of the American Medical Association - Surgery, September 2013, American Medical Association, www.jamanetwork.com; Jennifer Grauberger, BA et al, "Allegations of Failure to Obtain Informed Consent in Spinal Surgery Medical Malpractice Claims," Journal of the American Medical Association Surgery, June 2017, American Medical Association, www.jamanetwork.com.

[329] Kamini Kuchinad et al, "End-of-life care for glioblastoma multiforme (GBM) patients at a large

academic center," Journal of Clinical Oncology, May 20, 2017, American Society of Clinical Oncology, www.ascopubs.org; Leslie P. Scheunemann, MD, MPH et al, "Clinician-Family Communication About Patients' Values and Preferences in Intensive Care Units," Journal of Internal Medicine, April 1, 2019, American Medical Association, www.jamanetwork.com.

[330] Liam Davenport, "Is It Ever Okay to Lie to Your Cancer Patient?", Medscape, October 9, 2018, www.medscape.com.

[331] Robert Y. Lee, MD, MS et al, "Association of Physician Orders for Life-Sustaining Treatment With ICU Admission Among Patients Hospitalized Near the End of Life," Journal of the American Medical Association - Original Investigation, February 2020, American Medical Association, www.ama-assn.org; Ferdinando L. Mirarchi, DO, FAAEM, FACEP et al, "TRIAD XII – Are Patients Aware of and Agree With DNR or POLST Orders in Their Medical Records," Journal of Patient Safety, September 2019, www.journals.lww.com.

[332] Union Pacific Railway Company v. Botsford, 141 U.S. 250 (1891). Library of Congress, www.loc.gov.

[333] "Genetic Testing for Inherited Cancer Susceptibility Syndromes," National Cancer Institute, accessed January 8, 2021, www.cancer.gov; "Genetic Testing, Screening, and Prevention for People with a Strong Family History of Colorectal Cancer," American Cancer Society, accessed January 6, 2021, www.cancer.org; "Why might someone have a genetic consultation?," U.S. National Library of Medicine, National Institutes of Health, September 17, 2020, U.S. Department of Health and Human Services, www.medlineplus.gov.

[334] "How comedians Jeannie and Jim Gaffigan used humor to cope with a brain tumor," Better by Today, July 23, 2018, www.nbcnews.com.

CHAPTER THIRTEEN

[335] To Err Is Human: Building a Safer Health System, Institute of Medicine, November 1999, National Academy of Sciences, www.nap.edu.

[336] Daniel R. Neuspiel, MD, MPH, Chapter 288: Medical Errors, Adverse Events, and Patient Safety, Textbook of Pediatric Care, accessed April 30, 2021, American Academy of Pediatrics, www.aap.org; Working to Reduce Medication Errors, Food and Drug Administration, August 23, 2019, U.S. Department of Health and Human Services, www.fda.gov; Promoting Patient Safety / Code of Medical Ethics Opinion 8.6, American Medical Association, accessed January 30, 2021, www.ama-assn.org; Ethan D. Grober, MD, MEd and John M.A. Bohnen, MD, "Defining medical error," Canadian Medical Association, February 2005, www.www.cma.ca.

[337] Winta T. Mehtsun, MD, MPH et al, "Surgical never events in the United States," Surgery, December 18, 2012, www.surgjournal.com; Megan Knowles, "13 statistics on never events," Becker's Hospital Review, July 3, 2018, www.beckershospitalreview.com.

[338] "Americans' Experiences with Medical Errors and Views on Patient Safety," NORC at the University of Chicago and IHI/NPSF Lucian Leape Institute, September 2017, www.ihi.org; Iowa Patient Safety Study: Iowans' Views on Medical Errors / Iowa Patient Safety Study, Heartland Health Research Institute, June 2017, www.hhri.net; "The Public's Views on Medical Error in Massachusetts," Harvard School of Public Health, December 2014, Harvard University, www.psnet.ahrq.gov; David W. Newman-Toker et al, "Rate of diagnostic errors and serious misdiagnosis-related harms for major vascular events, infections, and cancers: toward a national incidence estimate using the 'Big Three'," Diagnosis, May 2020, Society to Improve Diagnosis in Medicine, www.degruyter.com; Hardeep Singh et al, "The frequency of diagnostic errors in outpatient care: estimations from three large observational studies involving US adult populations," BMJ Quality & Safety, April 17, 2014, www.bmj.com; Malpractice Risks in Communication Failures / 2015 CRICO Strategies National CBS Report, CRICO Strategies, The Risk Management Foundation of the Harvard Medical Institutions Incorporated, 2015, www.rmf.harvard.edu; Robert Hanscom, PhD et al, "A Dose of Insight / Diagnostic Accuracy: Room for Improvement," Coverys, April 2019, www.dashboard.coverys.com; Safe Surgery, Joint Commission Center for Transforming Healthcare, September 2, 2020, The Joint Commission, www.centerfortransforminghealthcare.org.

[339] "Americans' Experiences with Medical Errors and Views on Patient Safety," NORC at the University

of Chicago and IHI/NPSF Lucian Leape Institute, September 2017, www.ihi.org; "The Public's Views on Medical Error in Massachusetts," Harvard School of Public Health, December 2014, Harvard University, www.harvard.edu.; David P. Lind, MBA et al, "Medical Errors in Iowa: Prevalence and Patients' Perspectives," Journal of Patient Safety, September 2020, www.journalpatientsafety.com; The Financial and Human Cost of Medical Error, Betsy Lehman Center for Patient Safety, June 2019, www.betsylehmancenterma.gov; "Leadership to Improve Diagnosis: A Call to Action," Agency for Healthcare Research and Quality, June 2021, U.S. Department of Health and Human Services, www.ahrq.gov.

[340] Adverse Events, Near Misses, and Errors, Patient Safety Primer, Patient Safety Network, Agency for Healthcare Research and Quality, September 2019, U.S. Department of Health and Human Services, www.psnet.ahrq.gov.

[341] "Fast Facts on U.S. Hospitals, 2020," American Hospital Association, January 2020, www.aha.org.

[342] Martin A. Makary and Michael Daniel, "Medical error—the third leading cause of death in the US," The BMJ, May 3, 2016, Johns Hopkins University School of Medicine, www.bmj.com; John T. James, PhD, "A new, evidence-based estimate of patient harms associated with hospital care," Journal of Patient Safety, September 2013, www.journalpatientsafety.com.

[343] Leading Causes of Death, from Mortality in the United States, 2019, Data Brief No. 395, National Center for Health Statistics, Centers for Disease Control and Prevention, December 2020, U.S. Department of Health and Human Services, www.cdc.gov.

[344] Luke Slawomirski et al, "The Economics of Patient Safety: Strengthening a value-based approach to reducing patient harm at national level," Organisation for Economic Co-operation and Development, March 2017, www.oedc.org.

[345] Thomas L. Rodziewicz et al, "Medical Error Prevention," National Institutes of Health, January 2020, U.S. Department of Health and Human Services, www.ncbi.nlm.nih.gov; "Leadership to Improve Diagnosis: A Call to Action," Agency for Healthcare Research and Quality, June 2021, U.S. Department of Health and Human Services, www.ahrq.gov.

[346] "Preventing Medication Errors: A $21 Billion Opportunity," Compact Action Brief: A Roadmap For Increasing Value in Health Care, National Priorities Partnership, December 2010, National Quality Forum, www.qualityforum.org; Rayhan A. Tariq et al, "Medication Dispensing Errors and Prevention," StatPearls Publishing – NCBI Bookshelf, National Library of Medicine, National Institutes of Health, November 17, 2020, U.S. Department of Health and Human Services, www.ncbi.nlm.hih.gov.

[347] Improving Diagnosis in Health Care, Institute of Medicine, December 2015, National Academy of Sciences, www.nap.edu; Kerm Henriksen et al (AHRQ Patient Safety Team), "Challenges and opportunities from the Agency for Healthcare Research and Quality (AHRQ) research summit on improving diagnosis: a proceedings review," Agency for Healthcare Research and Quality, May 23, 2017, U.S. Department of Health and Human Services, www.ahrq.gov; "Leadership to Improve Diagnosis: A Call to Action," Agency for Healthcare Research and Quality, June 2021, U.S. Department of Health and Human Services, www.ahrq.gov; Hardeep Singh et al, "The frequency of diagnostic errors in outpatient care: estimations from three large observational studies involving US adult populations," BMJ Quality & Safety, April 17, 2014, www.bmj.com; David W. Newman-Toker et al, "Rate of diagnostic errors and serious misdiagnosis-related harms for major vascular events, infections, and cancers: toward a national incidence estimate using the 'Big Three'," Diagnosis, May 14, 2020, Society to Improve Diagnosis in Medicine, www.degruyter.com; Christina L. Cifra, "Diagnostic Errors in Pediatric Critical Care: A Systematic Review," Pediatric Critical Care Medicine, April 8, 2021, The Society of Critical Care Medicine and the World Federation of Pediatric Intensive and Critical Care Societies, www.journals.lww.com/pccmjournal.

[348] Elizabeth Zimmermann, "Mayo Clinic researchers demonstrate value of second opinions," Mayo Clinic, April 4, 2017, www.mayoclinic.org.

[349] James Mangan, RPh, "Top medication errors patients make at home," Becker's Hospital Review, July 10, 2019, www.beckershospitalreview.com.

[350] Erin J. Copi et al, "Evaluation of the frequency of dispensing electronically discontinued medications and associated outcomes," Journal of the American Pharmacists Association, July-August 2018, American Pharmacists Association, www.japha.org.

[351] Seth A. Seabury, PhD et al, "Assessment of Follow-up Care After Emergency Department Presentation for Mild Traumatic Brain Injury and Concussion / Results from the TRACK-TBI Study," JAMA Network Open, May 25, 2018, American Medical Association, www.jamanetwork.com.

[352] "Health Care-Associated Infections / Patient Safety Primer," Patient Safety Network, Agency for Healthcare Research and Quality, September 2019, U.S. Department of Health and Human Services, www.psnet.ahrq.gov; "Hospital-Acquired Conditions," Centers for Medicare and Medicaid Services, February 11, 2020, U.S. Department of Heath and Human Services, www.cms.gov; "Frequently Asked Questions – Deficit Reduction Act (DRA) Hospital-Acquired Condition (HAC) Reporting," Centers for Medicare and Medicaid Services, 2019, U.S. Department of Heath and Human Services, www.cms.gov.

[353] Mark R. Chassin, MD, FACP, MPP, MPH et al, "Improving Hand Hygiene at Eight Hospitals in the United States by Targeting Specific Causes of Noncompliance," The Joint Commission Journal on Quality and Patient Safety, January 2015, The Joint Commission, www.jointcommission.org; "Clean Hands Count for Safe Healthcare / What's the problem?," Centers for Disease Control and Prevention, March 15, 2016, U.S. Department of Health and Human Services, www.cdc.gov; Hand Hygiene, Joint Commission Center for Transforming Healthcare, accessed September 2, 2020, The Joint Commission, www.centerfortransforminghealthcare.org.

[354] Justification of Estimates for Appropriations Committees, FY 2020, Centers for Medicare and Medicaid Services, accessed December 26, 2020, U.S. Department of Health and Human Services, www.cms.gov; Preventing Pressure Ulcers in Hospitals, Agency for Healthcare Research and Quality, accessed January 28, 2021, U.S. Department of Health and Human Services, www.ahrq.gov.

[355] To Err Is Human: Building a Safer Health System, Institute of Medicine, November 1999, National Academy of Sciences, www.nap.edu.

[356] Kayhan Parsi, JD, PhD, "To Err is Human: Understanding the Data," AMA Journal of Ethics / Medicine and Society, March 2004, American Medical Association, www.journalofethics.ama-assn.org; "Medical Error – the third leading cause of death in the U.S.," Recorded interview with Martin A. Makary, MD on May 3, 2016, BMJ, www.bmj.com.

[357] National Healthcare Quality and Disparities Report, Agency for Healthcare Research and Quality, AHRQ Publication No. 20(21)-0045-EF, December 2020, U.S. Department of Health and Human Services, www.ahrq.gov; National Healthcare Quality and Disparities Report / Chartbook on Patient Safety, Agency for Healthcare Research and Quality, AHRQ Publication No. 21-0012, Updates 19(20)-0070-2-EF, February 2021, U.S. Department of Health and Human Services, www.ahrq.gov.

[358] Gopal Khanna, MBA, "After 20 Years of Improving America's Healthcare, AHRQ Makes Bold Plans for Future Successes," Agency for Healthcare Research and Quality, September 23, 2019, U.S. Department of Health and Human Services, www.ahrq.gov; "Leadership to Improve Diagnosis: A Call to Action," Agency for Healthcare Research and Quality, June 2021, U.S. Department of Health and Human Services, www.ahrq.gov.

[359] Sepsis – Clinical Information, Centers for Disease Control and Prevention, December 7, 2020, U.S. Department of Health and Human Services, www.cdc.gov; Adult, Nonmaternal Inpatient Stays Related to Sepsis: National Trends by Expected Primary Payer, 2012-2018, Healthcare Cost and Utilization Project, Agency for Healthcare Research and Quality, November 10, 2020, U.S. Department of Health and Human Services, www.ahrq.gov; Timothy G. Buchman, PhD, MD et al, "Sepsis Among Medicare Beneficiaries: 1. The Burdens of Sepsis, 2012-2018," Critical Care Medicine, March 2020, Society of Critical Care Medicine, www.ccmjournal.org.

[360] Surgical Site Infections, Patient Safety Primer, Patient Safety Network, Agency for Healthcare Research and Quality, September 2019, U.S. Department of Health and Human Services, www.psnet.ahrq.gov.

[361] The integrity of this statistic is in question, as every source concerning pressure ulcer fatalities since

1989 has been citing the same study from over three decades ago (Richard M. Allman, MD, "Pressure Ulcers among the Elderly," The New England Journal of Medicine, March 30, 1989, www.nejm.org), including the following: Justification of Estimates for Appropriations Committees, FY 2022, Centers for Medicare and Medicaid Services, May 3, 2021, U.S. Department of Health and Human Services, www.cms.gov; Preventing Pressure Ulcers in Hospitals, A Toolkit for Improving Quality of Care, Agency for Healthcare Research and Quality website, October 2014, accessed February 4, 2021, U.S. Department of Health and Human Services, www.ahrq.gov; Shawna Smith et al, "Success in Hospital-Acquired Pressure Ulcer Prevention: A Tail in Two Data Sets," Health Affairs, November 2018, Project HOPE, The People-to-People Health Foundation, Inc., www.healthaffairs.org; Christian N. Kirman, MD, "What is the mortality rate for pressure injuries (pressure ulcers)?," Medscape, March 26, 2020, www.medscape.com.

[362] Rayhan A. Tariq et al, "Medication Dispensing Errors and Prevention," StatPearls Publishing – NCBI Bookshelf, National Library of Medicine, National Institutes of Health, November 17, 2020, U.S. Department of Health and Human Services, www.ncbi.nlm.nih.gov.

[363] "Leadership to Improve Diagnosis: A Call to Action," Agency for Healthcare Research and Quality, June 2021, U.S. Department of Health and Human Services, www.ahrq.gov; Kerm Henriksen et al (AHRQ Patient Safety Team), "Challenges and Opportunities from the Agency for Healthcare Research and Quality (AHRQ) research summit on improving diagnosis: a proceedings review," Agency for Healthcare Research and Quality, May 23, 2017, U.S. Department of Health and Human Services, www.ahrq.gov; Percentage of Deaths, by Place of Death, National Vital Statistics System, United States, 2000-2018, Morbidity and Mortality Weekly Report, National Center for Health Statistics, Centers for Disease Control and Prevention, May 15, 2020, U.S. Department of Health and Human Services, www.cdc.gov; Deaths: Final Data for 2018, National Center for Health Statistics, Centers for Disease Control and Prevention, January 12, 2021, U.S. Department of Health and Human Services, www.cdc.gov; Improving Diagnosis in Health Care, Institute of Medicine, December 2015, National Academy of Sciences, www.nap.edu; Sarah H. Cross, MSW, MPH and Haider J. Warraich, MD, "Changes in the Place of Death in the United States," New England Journal of Medicine, December 12, 2019, Massachusetts Medical Society, www.nejm.org.

[364] To Err Is Human: Building a Safer Health System, Institute of Medicine, November 1999, National Academy of Sciences, www.nap.edu.

[365] Improving Diagnosis in Health Care, Institute of Medicine, December 2015, National Academy of Sciences, www.nap.edu.

[366] "Americans' Experiences with Medical Errors and Views on Patient Safety," NORC at the University of Chicago and IHI/NPSF Lucian Leape Institute, September 2017, www.ihi.org.

[367] Committee on Quality of Health Care in America, "To Err is Human: Building a Safer Health System," Institute of Medicine, November 1999, National Academy of Sciences, www.nap.edu.

[368] Kerm Henriksen et al (AHRQ Patient Safety Team), "Challenges and opportunities from the Agency for Healthcare Research and Quality (AHRQ) research summit on improving diagnosis: a proceedings review," Agency for Healthcare Research and Quality, May 23, 2017, U.S. Department of Health and Human Services, www.ahrq.gov.

[369] Mission and Budget, FY 2021 Budget [AHRQ], National Institutes of Health, National Institute for Research on Safety and Quality, February 2020, U.S. Department of Health and Human Services, www.ahrq.gov; National Institutes of Health (NIH) Funding: FY1995-FY2021, Congressional Research Services, May 12, 2020, www.crsreports.congress.gov.

[370] FY 2021 Budget Submission, Medical Programs and Information Technology Programs, Volume 2 of 4, U.S. Department of Veterans Affairs, February 2020, www.va.gov.

[371] Carrie Hanlon et al, 2014 Guide to State Adverse Event Reporting Systems, January 2015, National Academy for State Health Policy, www.nashp.org.

[372] State Government Tracking of Hospital-Acquired Conditions, RTI International, prepared for Centers for Medicare and Medicaid Services, June 2010, U.S. Department of Health and Human Services, www.cms.gov; Update on State Government Tracking of Health Care-Acquired Conditions and a Four-

State In-Depth Review – Final, RTI International, prepared for Centers for Medicare and Medicaid Services, June 2012, U.S. Department of Health and Human Services, www.cms.gov; Monitoring and Reporting Hospital-Acquired Conditions: A Federalist Approach, Medicare & Medicaid Research Review, Centers for Medicare and Medicaid Services, Office of Information Products & Data Analysis, 2014, U.S. Department of Health and Human Services, www.cms.gov; States with HAI Reporting Mandates, Centers for Medicare and Medicaid Services, November 13, 2019, accessed January 14, 2021, U.S. Department of Health and Human Services, www.cdc.gov.

[373] Improving Diagnosis in Health Care, Institute of Medicine, December 2015, National Academy of Sciences, www.nap.edu.

[374] Joseph Rencic, MD et al, "Clinical Reasoning Education at US Medical Schools: Results from a National Survey of Internal Medicine Clerkship Directors," Journal of General Internal Medicine, August 24, 2017, Society of General Internal Medicine, www.springer.com; Tejal K. Gandhi et al, "Transforming concepts in patient safety: a progress report," BMJ Open Access, June 2018, BMJ, www.qualitysafety.bmj.com; Mark L Graber, MD et al, "Improving diagnosis by improving education: a policy brief on education in healthcare professions," Diagnosis, August 27, 2018, Society to Improve Diagnosis in Medicine, www.degruyter.com.

[375] WHO Surgical Safety Checklist, World Health Organization, 2009, www.who.int; David L. Hepner, JD, MPh et al, "Operating Room Crisis Checklists and Emergency Manuals," Anesthesiology, August 2017, American Association of Anesthesiologists, www.pubs.asahq.org; "Checking on the Checklist," Lifebox and Ariadne Labs, 2020, www.lifebox.org.

[376] Angie Stewart, "Outpatient surgery growth over 15 years—12 statistics," Becker's ASC Review Newsletter, October 21, 2019, Becker's Ambulatory Surgery Center Review, www.beckersasc.com; Ambulatory Surgery Centers: Becoming Big Business, L.E.K. Insights, accessed January 29, 2021, L.E.K. Consulting, www.lek.com.

[377] "Hospital-Acquired Conditions," Centers for Medicare and Medicaid Services, February 11, 2020, U.S. Department of Heath and Human Services, www.cms.gov.

[378] "Update: MedPAC's Evaluation of Medicare's Hospital Readmission Reduction Program," MedPAC, the Medicare Payment Advisory Commission, December 2, 2019, www.medpac.gov; Jordan Rau, "New Round of Medicare Readmission Penalties Hits 2,583 Hospitals," Kaiser Health News, October 1, 2019, Kaiser Family Foundation, www.khn.org.

[379] Preventing Healthcare-associated Infections, Centers for Disease Control and Prevention, page last reviewed November 13, 2015, accessed January 29, 2021, U.S. Department of Health and Human Services, www.cdc.gov; Sepsis – Clinical Information, Centers for Disease Control and Prevention, December 7, 2020, U.S. Department of Health and Human Services, www.cdc.gov; Timothy G. Buchman, PhD, MD et al, "Sepsis Among Medicare Beneficiaries: 1. The Burdens of Sepsis, 2012-2018," Critical Care Medicine, March 2020, Society of Critical Care Medicine, www.ccmjournal.org.

[380] "Working Group Structure of the HAI Steering Committee," Steering Committee, Office of Disease Prevention and Health Promotion, accessed June 19, 2021, U.S. Department of Health and Human Services, www.health.gov; emails between the author and staff of Office of Infectious Disease and HIV/AIDS Policy under the Assistant Secretary for Health, January 27, 2021 – February 11, 2021.

[381] R. Monina Klevens, DDS, MPH et al, "Estimating Health Care-Associated Infections and Deaths in U.S. Hospitals, 2002," Public Health Reports, March-April 2007, www.hcbi.nlm.nih.gov; 4 Ways to Get Ahead of Sepsis, Centers for Disease Control and Prevention, September 1, 2020, www.cdc.gov; Aaron N. Dunn, BA et al, "Multidrug-resistant organisms on patients hands in an ICU setting," Infection Control & Hospital Epidemiology, February 2020, Cambridge University Press, www.cambridge.org.

[382] Justification of Estimates for Appropriations Committees, FY 2022, Centers for Medicare and Medicaid Services, May 3, 2021, U.S. Department of Health and Human Services, www.cms.gov; "Joint Commission Center for Transforming Healthcare, Leading Hospitals Partner to Reduce Hospital Acquired Pressure Injuries," Joint Commission Center for Transforming Healthcare, October 7, 2020, The Joint Commission, www.centerfortransforminghealthcare.org.

[383] "Americans' Experiences with Medical Errors and Views on Patient Safety," NORC at the University of Chicago and IHI/NPSF Lucian Leape Institute, September 2017, www.ihi.org.
[384] Gopal Khanna, MBA, "After 20 Years of Improving America's Healthcare, AHRQ Makes Bold Plans for Future Successes," Agency for Healthcare Research and Quality, September 23, 2019, U.S. Department of Health and Human Services, www.ahrq.gov.
[385] National Healthcare Quality and Disparities Report, Agency for Healthcare Research and Quality, AHRQ Publication 20(21)-0045-EF, December 2020, U.S. Department of Health and Human Services, www.ahrq.gov; National Healthcare Quality and Disparities Report / Chartbook on Patient Safety, Agency for Healthcare Research and Quality, AHRQ Publication No. 21-0012, Updates 19(20)-0070-2-EF, February 2021, U.S. Department of Health and Human Services, www.ahrq.gov; "Leadership to Improve Diagnosis: A Call to Action," Agency for Healthcare Research and Quality, June 2021, U.S. Department of Health and Human Services, www.ahrq.gov; "Indefinite Delivery Contract HHSP2332015000221," GovTribe, Inc., accessed June 24, 2021, www.govtribe.com.
[386] "AHRQ's Patient Safety Initiative: Building Foundations, Reducing Risk – Chapter 2. Efforts to Reduce Medical Errors: AHRQ's Response to Senate Committee on Appropriations Questions," Agency for Healthcare Research and Quality, 2003, accessed August 14, 2020, U.S. Department of Health and Human Services, www.ahrq.gov; Guide to Patient and Family Engagement in Hospital Quality and Safety, Agency for Healthcare Research and Quality, created September 2012, accessed August 14, 2020, U.S. Department of Health and Human Services, www.ahrq.gov.
[387] Peter Pronovost, Director, Johns Hopkins Hospital and Armstrong Institute for Patient Safety and Quality, introduction to online patient safety course, June 4, 2019, www.hopkinsmedicine.org.

CHAPTER FOURTEEN

[388] "Alzheimer's disease," Mayo Clinic, accessed August 22, 2020, www.mayoclinic.org; "2020 Alzheimer's Disease Facts and Figures," Alzheimer's & Dementia, Journal of the Alzheimer's Association, March 2020, Alzheimer's Association, www.alz.org; Subapriya Suppiah et al, "The Who, When, Why, and How of PET Amyloid Imaging in Management of Alzheimer's Disease—Review of Literature and Interesting Images," Diagnostics, June 25, 2019, www.mdpi.com; "Decision Memo for Beta Amyloid Positron Emission Tomography in Dementia and Neurodegenerative Disease (CAG-00431N)," Centers for Disease Control and Prevention, September 27, 2013, U.S. Department of Health and Human Services, www.cdc.gov.
[389] Sebastian Palmqvist, MD, PhD et al, "Discriminative Accuracy of Plasma Phospho-tau217 for Alzheimer Disease vs Other Neurodegenerative Disorders," Journal of the American Medical Association, July 28, 2020, American Medical Association, www.jamanetwork.com; "A Blood Test for Alzheimer's? Markers for Tau Take Us a Step Closer / Press Release," Alzheimer's Association International Conference, July 28, 2020, Alzheimer's Association, www.alz.org/aaic.
[390] Jim Atherton, MD, "Development of the Electronic Health Record," AMA Journal of Ethics, March 2011, American Medical Association, www.journalofethics.ama-assn.org; Percent of Hospitals, By Type, that Possess Certified Health IT, Office of the National Coordinator for Health Information Technology (ONC), September 2018, U.S. Department of Health and Human Services, www.healthit.gov; "EHR Incentive Program," Centers for Medicare and Medicaid Services, April 2018, U.S. Department of Health and Human Services, www.cms.gov.
[391] "Ways to Improve Electronic Health Record Safety," The PEW Charitable Trusts, American Medical Association & Medstar Health, August 2018, www.pewtrusts.org; Taking Action Against Clinician Burnout: A Systems Approach to Professional Well-Being, Committee on Systems Approaches to Improve Patient Care by Supporting Clinician Well-Being, 2019, National Academy of Medicine, www.nap.edu.
[392] Erika Fry and Fred Schulte, "Death By A Thousand Clicks," Fortune Magazine, April 1, 2019, Fortune and Kaiser Health News, www.fortune.com; Sigall K. Bell, MD et al, "Frequency and Types of Patient-Reported Errors in Electronic Health Ambulatory Care Notes," JAMA Network Open, June 9, 2020, American Medical Association, www.jamanetwork.com.

[393] David C. Classen, MD, MS et al, "National Trends in the Safety Performance of Electronic Health Record Systems From 2009 to 2018," JAMA Network Open, May 29, 2020, American Medical Association, www.jamanetwork.com; J. Marc Overhage, MD, PhD and Kevin B. Johnson, MD, MS, "Pediatrician Electronic Health Record Time Use for Outpatient Encounters," Pediatrics, December 2020, American Academy of Pediatrics, www.aappublications.org.
[394] "Health Care Professional EHR Health IT Developers," HealthIT Quick-Stat #30, Office of the National Coordinator for Health Information Technology (ONC), July 2017, U.S. Department of Health and Human Services, www.healthit.gov; Procuring Interoperability – Achieving High-Quality, Connected, and Person-Centered Care, National Academy of Medicine, 2018, www.nam.edu; Paul Warburton, "U.S. Hospital EMR Market Share 2019 Report," KLAS Research, April 30, 2019, www.klasresearch.com.
[395] Margaret Rouse, "FHIR (Fast Healthcare Interoperability Resources)," Tech Target, 2011, www.searchhealthit.techtarget.com; HL7 FHIR Release 4, FHIR Overview, Health Level Seven International, October 30, 2019, www.hl7.org; "About the ONC Health IT Certification Program," Office of the National Coordinator for Health Information Technology (ONC), July 20, 2020, U.S. Department of Health and Human Services, www.healthit.gov.
[396] Department of Health and Human Services, Centers for Medicare & Medicaid Services, Federal Register / Vol. 85, No. 85, Friday, May 1, 2020 / Rules and Regulations; Ben Moscovitch, "The public health case for federal health IT rules," The Hill, February 1, 2020, www.thehill.com; SHO #20-003 / Re: Implementation of the CMS Interoperability and Patient Access Final Rule and Compliance with the ONC 21st Century Cures Act Final Rule, Centers for Medicare and Medicaid Services, August 14, 2020, U.S. Department of Health and Human Services, www.cms.gov.
[397] "Part 1 and Part 2, What is information blocking?," American Medical Association, April 8, 2021, www.ama-assn.org; Jackie Drees, "HHS interoperability rules now in effect: 5 key compliance dates to know," Becker's Hospital Review, July 8, 2020, www.beckershospitalreview.com; "Cures Act Final Rule - Highlighted Regulatory Dates," Office of the National Coordinator for Health Information Technology, May 1, 2020, U.S. Department of Health and Human Services, www.healthit.gov.
[398] "Federal Requirements for Sharing Patient Medical Records Pose Major Challenges and Opportunities for Healthcare Organizations," Accenture U.S., October 15, 2019, www.accenture.com.
[399] Greg Slabodkin, "VA requests $2.6B in FY 2021 for Cerner EHR system," Health Data Management, February 10, 2020, www.healthdatamanagement.com; Hailey Mensik, "Rollout of VA's troubled Cerner EHR system delayed," HealthCareDive, February 12, 2020, www.healthcaredive.com; "VA Responds to COVID-19 with Schedule Revisions to Electronic Health Record Implementation," Department of Veterans Affairs, August 7, 2020, www.va.gov; Customer Experience Milestone: VA launches new Electronic Health Record System, email from U.S. Department of Veterans Affairs, October 28, 2020, www.va.gov.
[400] "Lifespan Pays $1,040,000 to OCR to Settle Unencrypted Stolen Laptop Breach," Office for Civil Rights, July 27, 2020, U.S. Department of Health and Human Services, www.hhs.gov.
[401] "Health Information Privacy - Breach Notification Rule," U.S. Department of Health and Human Services, July 26, 2013, accessed September 6, 2020, www.hhs.gov.
[402] "June 2019 Healthcare Data Breach Report," HIPAA Journal, July 24, 2019, www.hipaajournal.com; "2019 Healthcare Data Breach Report," HIPAA Journal, February 13, 2020, www.hipaajournal.com.
[403] "2020 Healthcare Data Breach Report: 25% Increase in Breaches in 2020," HIPAA Journal, January 19, 2021, www.hipaajournal.com; "Healthcare Data Breach Statistics," HIPAA Journal, January 8, 2021, www.hipaajournal.com.
[404] "A New In-Depth Analysis of Anthem Breach," Bank Info Security, January 10, 2017, www.bankinfosecurity.com.
[405] "Healthcare Data Breach Statistics," HIPAA Journal, January 8, 2021, www.hipaajournal.com.
[406] "2019 Healthcare Data Breach Report," HIPAA Journal, February 13, 2020, www.hipaajournal.com; Morgan Haefner, "Email hack exposes data of 485K Aetna, Blue Cross members," Becker's Hospital

Review, December 24, 2020, www.beckershospitalreview.com.

[407] "Blackbaud Data Breach Healthcare Victim Count Rises to Almost 1 Million," HIPAA Journal, September 4, 2020, www.hipaajournal.com; "Blackbaud security breach hits 11 systems: Atrium, NorthShore University, UK HealthCare & more," Becker's Hospital Review, September 9, 2020, www.beckershospitalreview.com; "Blackbaud Confirms Hackers Stole Some SSNs, as Lawsuits Increase," Health IT Security, September 30, 2020, www.healthitsecurity.com; "2020 Healthcare Data Breach Report: 25% Increase in Breaches in 2020," HIPAA Journal, January 19, 2021, www.hipaajournal.com.

[408] "Update: The 10 Biggest Healthcare Data Breaches of 2020, So Far," Health IT Security, July 8, 2020, www.healthitsecurity.com.

[409] Protecting Patient Information in the Age of Breaches, Health Information Management, accessed September 7, 2020, University of Illinois at Chicago, www.healthinformatics.uic.edu; Security Report: Health Care – Hospitals, Providers and more, Corvus Insurance, 2020, www.corvusinsurance.com.

[410] Ransomware Attacks Account for Almost Half of Healthcare Data Breaches," HIPAA Journal, January 28, 2021, www.hipaajournal.com

[411] "Information Breach on HealthCare.gov," Centers for Medicare and Medicaid Services, November 2018, U.S. Department of Health and Human Services, www.healthcare.gov; "Blue Button 2.0 API Update," Centers for Medicare and Medicaid Services, December 27, 2019, U.S. Department of Health and Human Services, www.bluebutton.cms.gov.

[412] Mackenzie Garrity, "Patient medical records sell for $1K on dark web," Becker's Hospital Review, February 20, 2019, www.beckerhospitalreview.com.

[413] Quinn Grundy et al, "Data sharing practices of medicines related apps and the mobile ecosystem: traffic, content, and network analysis," BMJ, March 20, 2019, www.bmj.com.

[414] Fred Bazzoli, "Epic to gather records of 20 million patients for medical research," Health Data Management, August 28, 2019, www.healthdatamanagement.com; Laura Dyrda, "5 Things to know about Epic's Cosmos," Becker's Hospital Review, September 8, 2020, www.beckershospitalreview.com; David Wahlberg, "Epic Systems records help find COVID-19 answers company is sharing online," Wisconsin State Journal, September 8, 2020, www.madison.com.

[415] Joyce E. Cutler, "How Can Patients Make Money Off Their Medical Data?" Pharmaceutical & Life Sciences News, January 29, 2019, Bloomberg Law, www.bloomberglaw.com.

[416] "Top 10 Technology Hazards for 2020," ECRI Institute, March 2020, www.ecri.org.

[417] "How doctors feel about Electronic Health Records," National Physician Poll by The Harris Poll, March 2018, Stanford Medical/Harris Poll, www.med.stanford.edu; Roger Collier, "Electronic health records contributing to physician burnout," Canadian Medical Association Journal, November 13, 2017, www.cmaj.ca; 2018 Survey of America's Physicians: Practice, Patterns and Perspectives, Physicians Foundation, September 2018, www.physiciansfoundation.org; The Future of Healthcare – A National Survey of Physicians – Electronic Health Records, The Doctors Company, Medical Malpractice Insurance, 2018, www.thedoctors.com.

[418] Taking Action Against Clinician Burnout: A Systems Approach to Professional Well-Being, Committee on Systems Approaches to Improve Patient Care by Supporting Clinician Well-Being, 2019, National Academy of Medicine, www.nap.edu; J. Marc Overhage and David McCallie, Jr., "Physician Time Spent Using the Electronic Health Record During Outpatient Encounters: A Descriptive Study," Annals of Internal Medicine, January 14, 2020, American College of Physicians, www.acpjournals.org; Sandra Scott Simons, MD, "Why EMRs Don't Work for EPs," Emerging Medicine News, January 2020, www.journals.lww.com.

[419] Mary Butler, "Finding John Doe: Patient Matching and the Need for a National Health Safety Identifier," Journal of AHIMA, March 2016, American Health Information Management Association, www.journal.ahima.org; "Harris County Hospital District Puts Patient Safety in the Palm of Your Hand," Harris County Hospital District, April 11, 2011, Harris Health System, www.prlog.org.

[420] Anuja Vaidya, "Top 10 Patient Safety Concerns for Healthcare Organizations 2020," ECRI Institute,

March 2020, www.ecri.org; Patient Identification and Matching Final Report, Office of the National Coordinator for Health Information Technology, February 7, 2014, U.S. Department of Health and Human Services, www.healthit.gov; ECRI Institute PSO Deep Dive: Patient Identification, ECRI Institute, September 28, 2016, www.ecri.org; Beth Haenke Just, MBA, RHIA, FAHIMA et al, "Why Patient Matching Is a Challenge: Research on Master Patient Index (MPI) Data Discrepancies in Key Identifying Fields," Perspectives in Health Information Management, April 1, 2016, American Health Information Management Association, www.perspectives.ahima.org; Erika Fry and Fred Schulte, "Death By A Thousand Clicks," Fortune Magazine, April 1, 2019, Fortune and Kaiser Health News, www.fortune.com; 2016 National Patient Misidentification Report, Ponemon Institute Research Report, December 2016, Ponemon Institute, www.imprivata.com.

[421] "Enhanced Patient Matching is Critical to Achieving Full Promise of Digital Health Records," The PEW Charitable Trusts, October 2, 2018, www.pewtrusts.org; Beth Haenke Just, MBA, RHIA, FAHIMA et al, "Why Patient Matching Is a Challenge: Research on Master Patient Index (MPI) Data Discrepancies in Key Identifying Fields," Perspectives in Health Information Management, April 1, 2016, American Health Information Management Association, www.perspectives.ahima.org.

[422] 2016 National Patient Misidentification Report, Ponemon Institute Research Report, December 2016, Ponemon Institute, www.imprivata.com.

[423] "HIPAA Background," Biological Sciences Division, HIPAA Program Office, October 23, 2006, University of Chicago, www.hipaa.bsd.uchicago.edu; Solomon I. Appavu, Analysis of Unique Patient Identifier Options – Final Report, prepared for The U.S. Department of Health and Human Services, November 24, 1997, www.hhs.gov; Richard Hillestad et al, "Identity Crisis – An Examination of the Costs and Benefits of a Unique Patient Identifier for the U.S. Health Care System," Rand Corporation, 2008, www.rand.org.

[424] Jessica Davis, "Congress Directs ONC to Support National Patient Identifier Efforts," Health IT Security, December 19, 2019, www.healthitsecurity.com; Letter to leaders of Senate Committee on Appropriations from 54 health care-related organizations seeking removal of ban on funding patient identifier adoption, August 27, 2019, www.strategichealthcare.net.

[425] Kate Monica, "National Patient Identifier Gains Congressional Support," EHRIntelligence, May 11, 2017, Extelligent Healthcare Media, www.ehrintelligence.com; Health Information Technology – Approaches and Challenges to Electronically Matching Patients' Records across Providers, Report to Congressional Committees, January 2019, United States Government Accountability Office, www.gao.gov; "Enhancing Patient Matching in Support of Operational Health Information Exchange (Indiana)," Agency for Healthcare Research and Quality, July 2017 to April 2022, U.S. Department of Health and Human Services, www.ahrq.gov; Patient Matching, Aggregation, and Linking Project – Final Report, Office of the National Coordinator of Health Information Technology, August 2019, U.S. Department of Health and Human Services, www.healthit.gov; "Patient Matching Algorithm Challenge," Challenge.gov, November 8, 2017, U.S. General Services Administration, www.challenge.gov.

[426] Taking Action Against Clinician Burnout: A Systems Approach to Professional Well-Being, Committee on Systems Approaches to Improve Patient Care by Supporting Clinician Well-Being, 2019, National Academy of Medicine, www.nap.edu.

[427] ECRI Institute PSO Deep Dive: Patient Identification, ECRI Institute Patient Safety Organization, August 2016, www.erci.org; Anuja Vaidya, "Top 10 Patient Safety Concerns for Healthcare Organizations 2020," ECRI Institute, March 2020, www.ecri.org; 2016 National Patient Misidentification Report, Ponemon Institute Research Report, December 2016, Ponemon Institute, www.imprivata.com.

[428] "What is telehealth? How is telehealth different from telemedicine?" Centers for Medicare and Medicaid Services, accessed August 24, 2020, U.S. Department of Health and Human Services, www.healthit.gov; "Telehealth and Telemedicine," American Academy of Family Physicians, July 2016, www.aafp.org; "Telemedicine Terms," Centers for Medicare and Medicaid Services, accessed September 1, 2020, U.S. Department of Health and Human Services, www.medicaid.gov.

[429] Kevin Ashton, "That 'Internet of Things' Thing," Radio Frequency Identification Journal, June 22,

2009, www.rfidjournal.com; Andrew Steger, "How the Internet of Medical Things (IoMT) Is Impacting Healthcare," HealthTech Magazine, January 16, 2020, www.healthtechmagazine.com; "Internet of Medical Things Revolutionizing Healthcare," Alliance of Advanced BioMedical Engineering, 2017, www.aabme.asme.org.

[430] Christopher Jason, "Google Digital Assistant Partnership Targets Physician Burnout," EHR Intelligence, October 31, 2019, xtelligent Healthcare Media, www.ehrintelligence.com.

[431] Jackie Drees, "Amazon's 1st wearable health tracker can share data directly with Cerner EHRs: 6 details," Becker's Hospital Review, August 27, 2020, www.beckershospitalreview.com; Joseph Goedert, "FDA clears wearable device to better monitor patients," Health Data Management, August 26, 2019, www.healthdatamanagement.com; "Smart Inhalers Market: An innovative solution for management of respiratory conditions," Biospace, April 8, 2020, www.biospace.com.

[432] "Increase Access to Health Assessment, Diagnosis, Care Delivery and Health Monitoring," Clinic-in-a-Bag, Rejuvin, accessed September 9, 2020, www.rejuvin.com.

[433] Lauren Smiley, "What Happens When We Let Tech Care for Our Aging Parents," WIRED, December 19, 2017, www.wired.com; "Care.Coach expands avatar deployments to fight COVID-19 loneliness epidemic," Business Insider, March 31, 2020, www.businessinsider.com.

[434] "Feeling sick? There's an app for that! – The Big Symptom Checker Review," The Medical Futurist, April 11, 2019, www.medicalfuturist.com.

[435] Taking Action Against Clinician Burnout: A Systems Approach to Professional Well-Being, Committee on Systems Approaches to Improve Patient Care by Supporting Clinician Well-Being, 2019, National Academy of Medicine, www.nap.edu; Jan Walker et al, "OpenNotes After 7 Years: Patient Experiences With Ongoing Access to Their Clinicians' Outpatient Visit Notes," Journal of Medical Internet Research, May 6, 2019, www.jmir.org; Vaishali Patel, MPH PhD and Christian Johnson, MPH, "Individuals' use of online medical records and technology for health needs," ONC Data Brief, Office of the National Coordinator for Health Information Technology, April 2018, U.S. Department of Health and Human Services, www.healthit.gov.

[436] Emily Guhl et al, "The Atrial Fibrillation Health Literacy Information Technology Trial: Pilot Trial of Mobile Health App for Atrial Fibrillation," Journal of Medical Internet Research – Cardio, September 4, 2020, www.cardio.jmir.org; Report to the Congress: Medicare and the Health Care Delivery System, Telehealth Services and the Medicare Program, Medicare Payment Advisory Commission, June 2016, www.medpac.gov; "Internet of Medical Things Revolutionizing Healthcare," Alliance of Advanced BioMedical Engineering, 2017, www.aabme.asme.org.

[437] "Evidence Reviews & Research Summaries," Centers for Disease Control and Prevention, accessed September 11, 2020, U.S. Department of Health and Human Services, www.cdc.com.

[438] Timothy W. Bickmore, PhD et al, "Patient and Consumer Safety Risks When Using Conversational Assistants for Medical Information: An Observational Study of Siri, Alexa, and Google Assistant," Journal of Medical Internet Research, September 2018, www.jmir.org; John Ferrand, MPH et al, "Evaluating Smart Assistant Responses for Accuracy and Misinformation Regarding Human Papillomavirus Vaccination Content Analysis Study," Journal of Medical Internet Research, August 2020, www.jmir.org.

[439] Nick Statt, "Boston Dynamics' Spot robot is helping hospitals remotely treat coronavirus patients," The Verge, April 23, 2020, www.theverge.com; "Work even better from anywhere," Double Robotics, accessed September 12, 2020, www.doublerobotics.com.

[440] Cynthia LeRouge and Monica J. Garfield, "Crossing the Telemedicine Chasm: Have the U.S. Barriers to Widespread Adoption of Telemedicine Been Significantly Reduced?," International Journal of Environmental Research and Public Health, December 2013, www.mdpi.com.

[441] June-Ho Kim et al, "How the Rapid Shift to Telehealth Leaves Many Community Health Centers Behind During The COVD-19 Pandemic," Project HOPE, The People-to-People Health Foundation, Inc., June 2, 2020, Health Affairs, www.healthaffairs.org; "Telemedicine," American Academy of Family Physicians, December 2019, www.aafp.org; "Virtual Visits: Telehealth and Older Adults," National Poll on Healthy Aging, October 2019, University of Michigan, www.healthyagingpoll.org.

[442] John D. Fanburg, JD and Jonathan J. Walzman, JD, "Telehealth and the law: the challenge of reimbursement," Medical Economics, September 12, 2018, www.medicaleconomics.com; State Telehealth Laws and Medicaid Program Policies, The Center for Connected Health Policy, Fall 2020, Public Health Institute, www.cchpca.org.
[443] "President Trump Expands Telehealth Benefits for Medicare Beneficiaries During COVID-19 Outbreak," Centers for Disease Control and Prevention, March 17, 2020, U.S. Department of Health and Human Services, www.cms.gov; "CMS Alert! Medicare Beneficiaries Expanded Telehealth Benefits During COVID-19 Outbreak," Telehealth Services, CMS Medical Learning Network, ICN MLN901705, March 2020, U.S. Department of Health and Human Services, www.cms.gov; Taylor Mallory Holland, "The new rules for remote patient monitoring reimbursement," Samsung Insights, September 2, 2020, www.insights.samsung.com; FDA News Release: Coronavirus (COVID-19) Update: FDA allows expanded use of devices to monitor patients' vital signs remotely, U.S. Food and Drug Administration, March 20, 2020, U.S. Department of Health and Human Services, www.fda.gov.
[444] Julie Hudman et al, "How Private Insurers Are Using Telehealth to Respond to the Pandemic," Health System Tracker, August 6, 2020, Peterson Center on Health Care – Kaiser Family Foundation, www.healthsystemtracker.org; Kara Gavin, "Telehealth Visits Skyrocket for Older Adults, but Concerns and Barriers Remain," University of Michigan M Health Lab, August 17, 2020, University of Michigan, www.labblog.uofmhealth.org; Jeff Rakeover et al, "Telemedicine: Center Quality and Safety," Institute for Healthcare Improvement, September/October 2020, www.ihi.org; Marc Zarefsky, "5 huge ways the pandemic has changed telemedicine," American Medical Association, August 26, 2020, www.ama-assn.org.
[445] Oleg Bestsennyy, "Telehealth: A quarter-trillion-dollar post-COVID-19 reality?," McKinsey & Company, May 29, 2020, www.mckinsey.com.
[446] "Trump Administration Finalizes Permanent Expansion of Medicare Telehealth Services and Improved Payment for Time Doctors Spend with Patients," Centers for Medicare and Medicaid Services, December 1, 2020, U.S. Department of Health and Human Services, www.cms.gov; 2020 Survey of America's Physicians / COVID-19 Impact Edition, Physicians Foundation, August 2020, www.physiciansfoundation.org.
[447] Ashish K. Khanna, MD et al, "The Multidisciplinary Critical Care Workforce: An Update from SCCM," Society of Critical Care Medicine, 2019, www.sccm.org.
[448] "Demographics of Internet and Home Broadband Usage in the United States," June 12, 2019, Pew Research Center, www.pewresearch.org.
[449] 2019 Broadband Deployment Report, Federal Communications Commission, May 8, 2019, www.fcc.gov; John Busby et al, "FCC Reports Broadband Unavailable to 21.3 Million Americans, BroadbandNow Study Indicates 42 Million Do Not Have Access," BroadbandNow Research, February 3, 2020, www.broadbandnow.com; John Kahan, "It's time for a new approach for mapping broadband data to better serve Americans," Microsoft on the Issues, April 8, 2019, Microsoft, www.microsoft.com.
[450] Cliff Coleman, MD, MPH, "Health Literacy and Clear Communication Best Practices for Telemedicine," Health Literacy Research and Practice, November 10, 2020, Healio, www.healio.com.
[451] "Future of Medicine, Telemedicine & Smartphones," The Medical Futurist, May 2, 2019, www.medicalfuturist.com; Third Annual Report – Final – Evaluation of Hospital-Setting HCIA Awards, Centers for Medicare and Medicaid Services, November 2, 2016, U.S. Department of Health and Human Services, www.cms.gov and www.abtassociates.com; Snigdha Jain, MD et al, "Availability of Telemedicine Services Across Hospitals in the United States in 2018: A Cross-sectional Study," Annals of Internal Medicine, April 30, 2020, American College of Physicians, www.acpjournals.org; Antonios Liolios, MD et al, "Working for a Remote Intensive Care Unit: How Does It Differ?," Medscape, March 18, 2019, www.medscape.com.
[452] Christian Millman, "10 Medical Advances That Will Shape the Future of Healthcare," Discover Magazine, October 23, 2019, www.discovermagazine.com; "Top 10 new medical technologies of 2019," Jahan Tajhiz Hakim Co., October 1, 2019, www.jahan-tajhiz.com; "Healthcare trends that will rock

medical care in the 2020s," Health Data Management, November 22, 2019, www.healthdatamanagement.com; "Artificial pancreas effectively controls type 1 diabetes in children age 6 and up," National Institutes of Health, August 26, 2020, U.S. Department of Health and Human Services, www.nih.gov; Monique Ellis, "Top 10 new medical technologies of 2019," Proclinical, February 27, 2019, www.proclinical.com; Rajni Setia, "An Overview of Ingestible Electronic Pills for Real-Time Analysis of Gastro-Intestinal Tract," Circuit Digest, February 25, 2020, www.circuitdigest.com; "Capsule Endoscopy (Pill Cam)," The Digestive Health Centre, accessed February 10, 2021, www.digestivehealth.com; "The Technological Future of Surgery," The Medical Futurist, January 17, 2017, www.medicalfuturist.com; Federica Cariati et al, "Innovative technologies for diagnosis and screening of genetic diseases in antenatal age, Journal of Laboratory and Precision Medicine, January 2020, www.jlpm.amegroups.com; Ahmed Hosny et al, "Artificial intelligence in radiology," Nature Reviews – Cancer, August 2018, www.nature.com; Ohad Oren, MD et al, "Artificial intelligence in medical imaging: switching from radiographic pathological data to clinically meaningful endpoints," The Lancet – Digital Health, September 2020, www.thelancet.com.

[453] Joel Berg, "You may think you've seen this telemedicine kiosk movie before but...," Med City News, October 17, 2019, www.medcitynews.com; "Telehealth Kiosks, American Well, accessed September 14, 2020, www.business.amwell.com.

[454] "Telestroke (stroke telemedicine)," Mayo Clinic, accessed September 9, 2020, www.mayoclinic.org; Webster Brehm, "How Telestroke Technology is Saving Lives (and Brains): Parts 1 of 2," American Well, June 13, 2017, www.business.amwell.com; Raghu Seethala, MD, "A Brief Review of Telemedicine in Critical Care," American College of Emergency Physicians, April 2017, www.acep.org.

[455] H.R. 4302 - Protecting Access to Medicare Act of 2014, Public Law No. 113-93, April 1, 2014, www.congress.gov; "Appropriate Use Criteria for Advanced Diagnostic Imaging," Medicare Learning Network, Centers for Medicare and Medicare, December 2018, U.S. Department of Health and Human Services, www.cms.gov.

[456] "Reporting appropriate use criteria in claims for Medicare patients," American Medical Association, accessed September 16, 2020, www.ama-assn.org; White Paper: Implementing a Successful AUC and CDSM Strategy for Advanced Imaging Procedures, Infinx Healthcare, July 2020, www.infinx.com; "Appropriate Use Criteria Program," Centers for Medicare and Medicaid Services, August 12, 2020, U.S. Department of Health and Human Services, www.cms.gov; "Clinical Decision Support Mechanisms," Centers for Medicare and Medicaid Services, August 10, 2020, U.S. Department of Health and Human Services, www.cms.gov.

[457] Emily Miller, "Types of Medical Device Applications," Drug Watch, April 21, 2020, www.drugwatch.com; "Step 3: Pathway to Approval," U.S. Food and Drug Administration, February 9, 2018, U.S. Department of Health and Human Services, www.fda.gov; Kyle H. Sheetz, MD, MSc et al, "Trends in the Adoption of Robotic Surgery for Common Surgical Procedures," JAMA Network Open, January 2020, American Medical Association, www.jamanetwork.com; Gail A. Van Norman, MD, "Drugs, Devices, and the FDA: Part 2: An Overview of Approval Processes: FDA Approval of Medical Devices," Journal of the American College of Cardiology, June 2016, American College of Cardiology, www.sciencedirect.com.

CHAPTER FIFTEEN

[458] Craig M. Hales, MD, MPH et al, "Prescription Drug Use Among Adults Aged 40-79 in the United States and Canada," National Center for Health Statistics, Centers for Disease Control and Prevention, August 2019, U.S. Department of Health and Human Services, www.cdc.gov; Medicine Use and Spending in the U.S. – A Review of 2018 and Outlook to 2023, IQVIA Institute for Human Data Science, May 2019, www.iqvia.com.

[459] Medicine Use and Spending in the U.S. – A Review of 2018 and Outlook to 2023, IQVIA Institute for Human Data Science, May 2019, www.iqvia.com; National Health Expenditures Fact Sheet, Historical NHE, 2019, U.S. Centers for Medicare and Medicaid Services, December 16, 2020, U.S. Department of Health and Human Services, www.cms.gov.

[460] J. Mark Ruscin, PharmD, FCCP, BCPS and Sunny A. Linnebur, PharmD, BCPS, BCGP, "Aging and Drugs," Merck Manuals Professional Edition, December 2018, Merck & Company, Inc., www.merckmanuals.com; J. Mark Ruscin, PharmD, FCCP, BCPS and Sunny A. Linnebur, PharmD, BCPS, BCGP, "Overview of Drug Therapy in Older Adults," Merck Manuals Professional Edition, December 2018, Merck & Company, Inc., www.merckmanuals.com.

[461] "Health Care Access and Utilization / Prescription Drugs," Health, United States – 2018, Centers for Disease Control and Prevention, October 30, 2019, U.S. Department of Health and Human Services, www.cdc.gov; "Adverse Drug Events: Magnitude of the Problem," National Action Plan for Adverse Drug Event Prevention, Office of Disease Prevention and Health Promotion, 2014, accessed March 8, 2021, U.S. Department of Health and Human Services, www.health.gov.

[462] Jonathan H. Watanabe, PharmD, MS, PhD et al, "Cost of Prescription Drug-Related Morbidity and Mortality," Annals of Pharmacotherapy, March 26, 2018, www.journals.sagepub.com.

[463] "Adverse Drug Events," Centers for Disease Control and Prevention, accessed September 30, 2020, U.S. Department of Health and Human Services, www.cdc.gov.

[464] Katie J. Quinn and Nigam H. Shah, "A dataset quantifying polypharmacy in the United States," Scientific Data, October 31, 2017, www.nature.com.

[465] Matthew Bledsoe, PharmD, MCPS, "Polypharmacy in the Elderly," Presentation at the Tennessee Center for Patient Safety, May 14, 2019, www.tnpatientsafety.com; "Medication Errors and Adverse Drug Events," Patient Safety Network, Agency for Healthcare Research and Quality, January 2019, U.S. Department of Health and Human Services, www.psnet.ahrq.gov.

[466] Adverse Drug Events, Adverse Drug Reactions and Medication Errors – Frequently Asked Questions, VA Center for Medication Safety, November 2006, Veterans Administration Center for Medication Safety, www.pbm.va.gov; Jamie J. Coleman and Jennifer K. Pontefract, "Adverse drug reactions," Clinical Medicine, October 2016, Royal College of Physicians, www.rcpjournals.org; "Preventable Adverse Drug Reactions: A Focus on Drug Interactions / FDA," U.S. Food and Drug Administration, March 6, 2018, accessed March 9, 2021, U.S. Department of Health and Human Services, www.fda.gov.

[467] Rayhan A. Tariq et al, "Medication Dispensing Errors and Prevention," StatPearls Publishing – NCBI Bookshelf, National Library of Medicine, National Institutes of Health, November 17, 2020, U.S. Department of Health and Human Services, www.ncbi.nlm.hih.gov.

[468] "Report: Two in Five Antibiotic Rxs May Not Be Needed," American Association of Family Practitioners, January 28, 2020, www.aafp.org; "Brain Bleed, Hemorrhage (Intracranial Hemorrhage)," Cleveland Clinic, accessed May 4, 2020, www.clevelandclinic.org.

[469] J. Mark Ruscin, PharmD, FCCP, BCPS and Sunny A. Linnebur, PharmD, BCPS, BCGP, "Aging and Drugs," Merck Manuals Professional Edition, December 2018, Merck & Company, Inc. www.merckmanuals.com; J. Mark Ruscin, PharmD, FCCP, BCPS and Sunny A. Linnebur, PharmD, BCPS, BCGP, "Pharmacokenetics in Older Adults," Merck Manuals Professional Edition, December 2018, Merck & Company, Inc., www.merckmanuals.com; Health Care Access and Utilization / Prescription Drugs, Health, United States – 2018, Centers for Disease Control and Prevention, October 30, 2019, U.S. Department of Health and Human Services, www.cdc.gov; Paula A. Rochon, MD, MPH, FRPC, "Drug prescribing for older adults," Wolters Kluwer Up to Date, June 8, 2020, www.uptodate.com; Jennifer Abbasi, "Older Patients (Still) Left Out of Cancer Clinical Trials," Medical News & Perspectives, Journal of the American Medical Association, October 24, 2019, American Medical Association, www.jamanetwork.com.

[470] Avantika A. Saraf et al, "Medications Associated with Geriatric Syndromes and Their Prevalence in Older Hospitalized Adults Discharged to Skilled Nursing Facilities," Journal of Hospital Medicine, June 3, 2016, Society of Hospital Medicine, www.journalofhospitalmedicine.com; Dima Mazen Qato et al, "Prevalence of Prescription Medications With Depression as a Potential Adverse Effect Among Adults in the United States," Journal of the American Medical Association, June 12, 2018, American Medical Association, www.jamanetwork.com.

[471] "Reporting Serious Problems to FDA," U.S. Food and Drug Administration, accessed October 1, 2020,

U.S. Department of Health and Human Services, www.fda.gov; "Working to Reduce Medication Errors," U.S. Food and Drug Administration, August 23, 2019, U.S. Department of Health and Human Services, www.fda.gov.
[472] Deep Dive: Safe Ambulatory Care, Patient Safety Organization, 2019, ECRI Institute, www.ecri.org.
[473] Patrick Viet-Quoc Nguyen, BPharm, MSc and Caroline Spinelli, "Prescribing cascade in an elderly woman," Canadian Pharmacists Journal, May 2016, Canadian Pharmacists Association, www.journals.sagepub.com.
[474] Matthew Bledsoe, PharmD, MCPS, "Polypharmacy in the Elderly," Presentation at the Tennessee Center for Patient Safety, May 14, 2019, www.tnpatientsafety.com.
[475] "Medication Errors: Cut your risk with these tips," Mayo Clinic, September 3, 2020, www.mayoclinic.org; "Working to Reduce Medication Errors," U.S. Food and Drug Administration, August 23, 2019, U.S. Department of Health and Human Services, www.fda.gov; 20 Tips to Help Prevent Medical Errors: Patient Fact Sheet," Agency for Healthcare Research and Quality, May 2017, U.S. Department of Health and Human Services, www.ahrq.gov.
[476] Chong-Han Kua, BSc (Pharm) et al, "Health Outcomes of Deprescribing Interventions Among Older Residents in Nursing Homes: A Systemic Review and Meta-analysis," Journal of the American Medical Directors Association, December 2018, The Society for Post-Acute and Long-Term Care Medicine, www.sciencedirect.com.

CHAPTER SIXTEEN

[477] Joint Commission Center for Transforming Healthcare Releases Targeted Solutions Tool for Hand-Off Communications, Joint Commission on Accreditation of Healthcare Organizations, August 2012, www.jointcommission.org; John W. Rusher, MD, JD, FAAP, "Improve patient handoffs to prevent medical errors, reduce malpractice risk," AAP News, January 9, 2020, The American Academy of Pediatrics, www.aappublications.org.
[478] "Inadequate hand-off communication," Sentinel Event Alert, September 12, 2017, The Joint Commission, www.jointcommission.org.
[479] "Does Your EMS-ED Handoff Process Need a Hand?," General Devices, January 23, 2020, www.openpr.com.
[480] E. Michael Lewiecki et al, "Challenges in osteoporosis awareness and management: results from a survey of U.S. postmenopausal women," Presented at the American Association of Nurse Practitioners 2018 National Conference, June 26-29, 2018, Clinical Advisor, www. clinicaladvisor.com.
[481] "Transitions of Care: Managing medications," Quick Safety / An advisory on safety & quality issues, Division of Health Care Improvement, August 2016, The Joint Commission, www.jointcommission.org.
[482] A. P. Tully et al, "Evaluation of medication errors at the transition of care from an ICU to non-ICU location," Patient Safety Network, Agency for Healthcare Research and Quality, January 2019, U.S. Department of Health and Human Services, www.psnet.ahrq.gov.
[483] Alok Kapoor, MD, MSc et al, "Adverse Events in Long-term Care Residents Transitioning from Hospital Back to Nursing Home," JAMA Internal Medicine, July 22, 2019, American Medical Association, www.jamainternalmedicine.com.
[484] "Inadequate hand-off communication," Sentinel Event Alert, September 12, 2017, The Joint Commission, September 12, 2017, www.jointcommission.org; Amit Prasad, MD et al, "Standardization Improves Postoperative Patient Handoff Experience for Junior Clinicians," American Journal of Managed Care, June 2020, www.ajmc.com; Abulaziz M. Saleem, MD et al, "Initial assessment of patient handoff in accredited general surgery residency programs in the United States and Canada: a cross-sectional survey," Canadian Journal of Surgery, August 2015, www.canjsurg.ca; Robyn Davis et al, "Patient Handoff Education: Are Medical Schools Catching up?," American Journal of Medical Quality, March/April 2018, American College of Medical Quality, www.us.sagepub.com.
[485] Adriana Hada and Finoa Coyer, "Shift-to-shift nursing handover interventions associated with improved inpatient outcomes—Falls, pressure injuries and medication administration errors: An integrative review," Nursing & Health Sciences, March 4, 2021, Wiley Online Library,

www.onlinelibrary.wiley.com; Jennifer L. W. Fink, BSN, "How Hospitalists Can Improve Shift-to-Shift Patient Handoffs," Medscape, January 18, 2019, www.medscape.com; Amy J. Starmer et al, "I-PASS, a Mnemonic to Standardize Verbal handoffs," Pediatrics, January 9, 2012, American Academy of Pediatrics, www.ipassinstitute.com.

[486] "What is a hospitalist? Guidelines for Communicating With the Referring Primary Care Physician," American Academy of Family Physicians, 2018, www.aafp.org.

[487] Valuation of Care Management Performed by Primary Care Physicians / An Issue Brief, American Academy of Family Physicians, May 2016, www.aafp.org; John Schurrer et al, Evaluation of the Diffusion and Impact of the Chronic Care Management (CCM) Services: Final Report, Center for Medicare and Medicaid Innovation, Center for Medicare and Medicaid Services, November 2, 2017, U.S. Department of Health and Human Services, www.cms.gov; Roberta Capp et al, "Coordination Program Reduced Acute Care Use and Increased Primary Care Visit Among Frequent Emergency Care Users," Health Affairs, October 2017, Project HOPE, The People-to-People Health Foundation, Inc., www.healthaffairs.org.

[488] Benefits of NCQA Patient-Centered Medical Home Recognition, National Committee for Quality Assurance, June 2019, www.ncqa.org; Susannah Higgins, MS et al, "Medical Homes and Costs and Utilization Among High-Risk Patients," American Journal of Managed Care, March 24, 2014, www.ajmc.com.

[489] Joint Principles of the Patient-Centered Medical Home, American Academy of Family Physicians et al, March 2007, www.acp.org; "The Medical Home – Five Key Functions of a Medical Home," American Academy of Family Physicians, accessed September 6, 2020, www.aafp.org; "Features of the Medical Home," Patient-Centered Primary Care Collaborative, accessed May 13, 2020, www.pcpcc.org.

[490] "Hidden Hazards: Closing the Care Gap Between Physicians and Patients With Multiple Chronic Conditions," Regina Corso Consulting on behalf of Quest Diagnostics, February 2018, www.questdiagnostics.com; Sumit D. Agarwal, MD et al, "Adoption of Medicare's Transitional Care Management and Chronic Care Management Codes in Primary Care," Journal of the American Medical Association, December 25, 2018, American Medical Association, www.jama.com; Providing and Billing Medicare for Chronic Care Management Services, PYA, PC, February 2020, www.pyapc.com; Fred Charatan, "U.S. Doctors Call for Simple Medicare Rules," BMJ, March 17, 2001, www.bmj.com.

[491] "Delivering Value-based Transformation in Primary Care, Centers for Medicare and Medicaid Services," April 22, 2019, U.S. Department of Health and Human Services, www.cms.gov; Jacqueline LaPointe, "Advanced Alternative Payment Model Participation Rose in 2018," Revenue Cycle Management, January 6, 2020, Xtelligent Healthcare Media, www.revcycleintelligence.com; "Evaluation of the Comprehensive Primary Care Plus Initiative (CPC+) / First Annual Report," Centers for Medicare and Medicaid Services, April 2019, U.S. Department of Health and Human Services, www.cms.gov; "Comprehensive Primary Care Plus (CPC+) Model / Evaluation of Second Year (2018)," Centers for Medicare and Medicaid Services, July 2020, U.S. Department of Health and Human Services, www.cms.gov; "Comprehensive Primary Care Plus," Centers for Medicare and Medicaid Services, October 6, 2020, U.S. Department of Health and Human Services, www.cms.gov; "Comprehensive Primary Care Plus (CPC+) Model / Evaluation of the Third Year (2019)," Centers for Medicare and Medicaid Services, January 2021, U.S. Department of Health and Human Services, www.cms.gov.

[492] Kelly Gooch, "CMS blasted for nearly 2-year delay in payout of Medicare performance bonuses," Becker's Hospital Review, September 18, 2019, www.beckershospitalreview.com; Quality Payment Program, Centers for Medicare and Medicaid Services, September 28, 2020, U.S. Department of Health and Human Services, www.cms.gov.

[493] Joint Commission Center for Transforming Healthcare Releases Targeted Solutions Tool for Hand-Off Communications, The Joint Commission, August 2012, www.jointcommission.org.

[494] Ernest Shen, PhD et al, "Association of a Dedicated Post-Hospital Discharge Follow-up Visit and 30-Day Readmission Risk in a Medicare Advantage Population," JAMA Internal Medicine, January 2017, American Medical Association, www.jamanetwork.com.

[495] Roberta Capp et al, "Assessing the Impact of Patient Navigation on Reducing Emergency Department

Visits for Adult Medicaid Frequent ED Users: A Randomized Control Trial," Annual Research Meeting, June 16, 2015, Academy Health, www.academyhealth.org.

[496] Alisa Khan, "Patient safety after implementation of a coproduced family centered communication programme: multicenter before and after interventions study," BMJ Open Access, October 2018, www.bmjopen.bmj.com.

A FEW CLOSING REMARKS

[497] Letter from Phillip L. Swagel, Director of the Congressional Budget Office to the Honorable Kevin McCarthy, Republican Leader, U.S. House of Representatives, Congressional Budget Office, February 25, 2021, www.cbo.gov; Kevin B. O'Reilly, "Biden signs bill delaying 2% Medicare sequester pay cut until 2022," Medicare & Medicaid, April 15, 2021, American Medical Association, www.ama-assn.org.

[498] "What We Know—and What We Don't Know—About the Impact of the Pandemic on Our Most Vulnerable Community," The COVID Tracking Project, accessed May 15, 2021, www.covidtracking.com.

[499] "Long-Term Care Ombudsman Program" (2016 data), Administration for Community Living, accessed June 13, 2021, U.S. Department of Health and Human Services, www.acl.gov; "The Long-Term Care Ombudsman Program," National Ombudsman Resource Center, February 12, 2020, www.ltcombudsman.org.

[500] "The Current ADA Regulations," Information and Technical Assistance on the Americans with Disabilities Act, Civil Rights Division, accessed May 13, 2021, U.S. Department of Justice, www.ada.gov; "Disability and Functioning," Centers for Disease Control and Prevention, accessed May 13, 2021, U.S. Department of Health and Human Services, www.cdc.gov.

[501] Jeff LaGasse, "Health literacy seen as an important tool in increasing COVID-19 vaccine uptake," Health Care Finance News, April 8, 2021, www.healthcarefinancenews.com.

[502] "Keep on Your Feet – Preventing Older Adult Falls," Injury Prevention & Control, Centers for Disease Control and Prevention, accessed June 8, 2021, U.S. Department of Health and Human Services, www.cdc.gov.

ABOUT THE AUTHOR

Jo Kline, J.D.

Jo Kline is an attorney, an expert on health literacy and a tireless advocate for patients' rights. She is also a Baby Boomer. Like many of her followers and readers, she became interested in the issue of medical decision making after witnessing a loved one's end of life. Soon after, while serving as volunteer chair of Iowa's largest hospice, Jo began to research, speak and write about the crucial role of advocacy in health care decision making. That was over 20 years ago. Much later, it was Jo's own medical crisis that taught her what it means to be truly *health literate*, and that led her to recognize the perfect storm threatening access to and delivery of health care in America.

When Jo began to write **Patient or Pawn?**, her mission was simple. First, to explore and reveal the demographics of aging and chronic illness that threaten patient rights to consent, autonomy and safety; and second, to share the health literacy strategies needed for self-preservation. More than 500 scholarly and statistical resources later, that's exactly what she has done.

Jo is also the author of **The Practical Guide to Health Care Advance Directives**, **The 60-Minute Guide to Health Literacy** and the award-winning **SO GROWS THE TREE – Creating an Ethical Will**. Among other print, online and broadcast media, Jo has been featured in *The New York Times*, *Reader's Digest*, *The Philadelphia Inquirer* and *The Des Moines Register*. She is a contributor to online news outlets, a frequent guest essayist for *The Des Moines Register* and the author of its ten-week series *Health Literacy 101*.

www.JoKline.net

Jo's email: PatientOrPawn@outlook.com

Made in the USA
Monee, IL
05 November 2026

67811478R20118